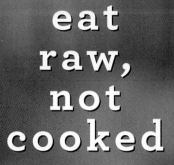

eat
raw,
not
cooked

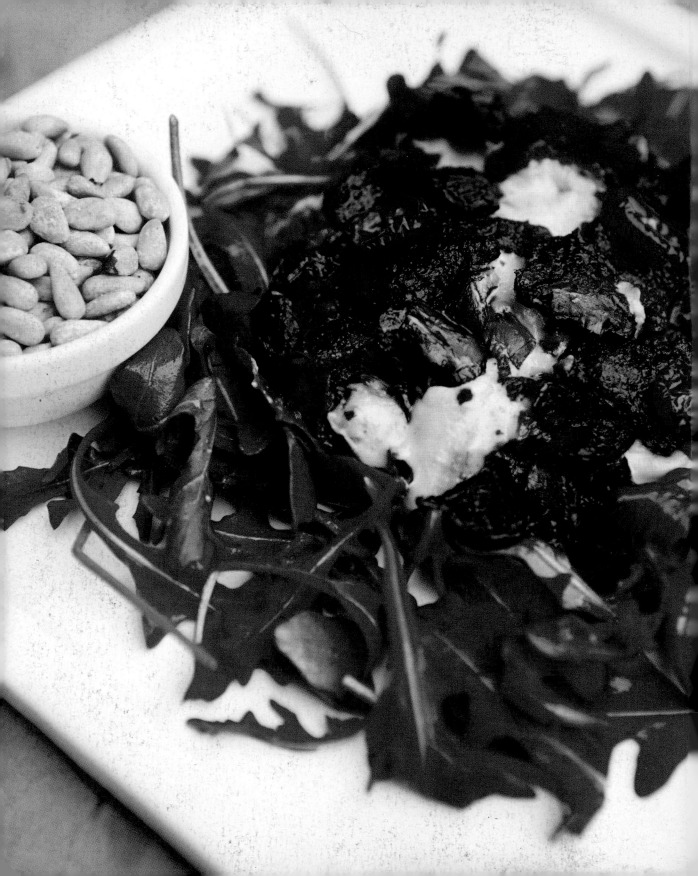

eat raw, not cooked

WITHDRAWN

STACY STOWERS

GALLERY BOOKS

new york ▪ london ▪ toronto ▪ sydney ▪ new delhi

G

Gallery Books
Division of Simon & Schuster, Inc.
1230 Avenue of the Americas
New York, NY 10020

Photographs © 2013 by Karen Nickel
Photographs on pages viii, xxvi, 2, 4, 6, 7, and 191 by Eli Dagostino

First Gallery Books trade paperback edition April 2014

GALLERY BOOKS and colophon are registered trademarks of Simon & Schuster, Inc.

For information about special discounts for bulk purchases, please contact Simon & Schuster Special Sales at 1-866-506-1949 or business@simonandschuster.com.

The Simon & Schuster Speakers Bureau can bring authors to your live event. For more information or to book an event contact the Simon & Schuster Speakers Bureau at 1-866-248-3049 or visit our website at www.simonspeakers.com.

Interior design by Jaime Putorti

Manufactured in the United States of America

10   9   8   7   6   5   4   3   2   1

Library of Congress Cataloging-in-Publication Data
Stowers, Stacy.
Eat raw, not cooked / Stacy Stowers.
    pages   cm
1. Raw foods. 2. Cooking (Vegetables) 3. Raw food diet—Recipes. I. Title.
TX742.S765 2014
613.2'65—dc23 2013040351

ISBN 978-1-4767-5207-5
ISBN 978-1-4767-5211-2 (ebook)

This book is dedicated to

all the families who feed my soul.

This is for you!

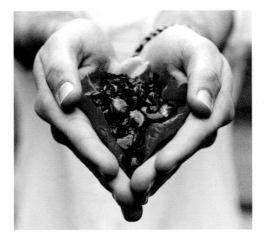

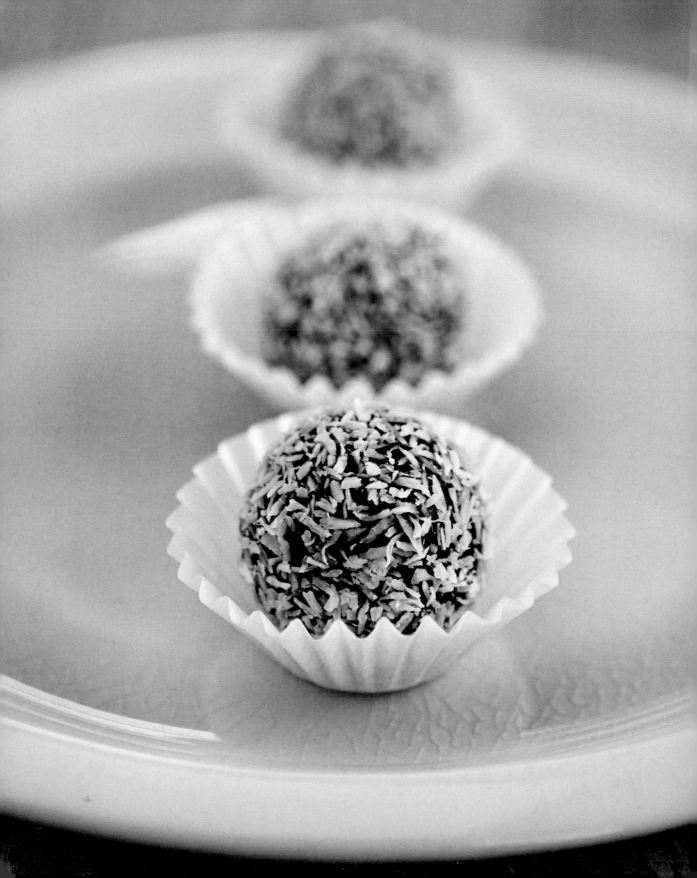

Contents

I was disabled for 17 years. My suffering ended in ten days when I did two things: I stopped cooking my food and I eliminated processed foods.
—Stacy Stowers

Introduction

As a society, we have become disconnected from our food, opting for the convenience of so many boxed, bagged, packaged, and bottled processed foods to accommodate our ever-demanding responsibilities and schedules. Nutrition is a complex field with conflicting theories about food continually up for debate. Yet despite all these theories in question, there are two things about nutrition that I believe absolutely to be true:

1. We must let go of processed foods.
2. Raw food heals.

Eat Raw, Not Cooked is a guide to introduce families to the pleasures of eating clean, rich, real food in its raw state. Since January 1, 2010, I have been traveling the country, living with a new family each week, with the goal of feeding and teaching people of all ages and backgrounds how to add more whole, raw, unprocessed foods to their diets and to do it in the simplest and most satisfying way possible. Through photographs, stories, and recipes, *Eat Raw, Not Cooked* follows my path across America from home to home, sharing the joy of these delicious healing foods with families of all kinds. Good nutrition has never been so easy or tasted this good!

These raw re-creations are not only flavorsome and satisfying, but also fast and easy—the recipes are simple, made from ingredients available in local markets . . . or at least a mouse click away. Welcome to a whole new way of enjoying your old favorite comfort foods.

▪ MY RAW STORY ▪

"There is nothing in a caterpillar that
tells you it is going to be a butterfly."
—Buckminster Fuller

"Let food be thy medicine,
and medicine be thy food."
—Hippocrates

I came to raw food reluctantly. I was comfortable with the convenience of my boxed, bottled, canned, bagged, frozen dinners. "Fat Free," "Sugar Free," and "Low Calorie" were the only labels I read on packages. I was the Microwave Bandit!

I looked good on the outside, but I was dying on the inside, literally. In the spring of 2007 at 39 years old, I found myself in bed, in pain, and on an array of medications, pain pills, sleeping pills, antidepressants, coffee, and alcohol. My personal life was an unmanaged wreck. My teeth eventually began to crack and fall out. It was then that I discovered raw food—albeit reluctantly. My life was about to change drastically—more dramatically than I could ever have imagined.

Before discovering raw foods, I had struggled with chronic pain and fatigue, ever since I was stricken at the age of 22 with valley fever, a fungal infection that attacks the body's immune system. In 2013, the *New York Times* described valley fever (coccidioidomycosis) as a "disease without a cure." After just ten days of eating my food raw and unprocessed, I started feeling better! My head was no longer foggy and the pain in my body: gone. I immediately went to work learning everything I could about raw food.

My heart burned to share my story throughout our country. If eating raw foods helped me so dramatically, perhaps it could help others. By January 1, 2010, I had sold everything I owned and took to the road on a one-year mission of sharing my story. My tour was so successful that families began emailing me from all parts of the country to please come teach them how to prepare raw food that tastes good—food the whole family would enjoy.

Now, from my home base in New York City, I continue to travel, providing families with a one-week full-immersion course into the flavors of our earth's most healing foods. Together, we re-create their favorite dishes. Yes, some family members are often reluctant, but once they taste the food, there's no denying the deliciousness—the proof is in the chocolate mousse.

▪ WHY EAT RAW FOOD? ▪

Because raw foods are good for you!

Eating a lot of raw food is key to any healthy diet. Raw fruits and vegetables are nutrient-rich and low in calories, which makes them ideal components of an anticancer diet and a healthy diet in general. High heat destroys the integrity of the nutrients found in raw foods, and toxic compounds (such as acrylamides) form, especially when frying or barbecuing. Eating our food in its original raw state is necessary for digestive efficiency and normal bowel function. Avocados, fruits, and nuts significantly change when you cook them and are at their very best when eaten raw. Cruciferous vegetables (broccoli, cauliflower, cabbage, kale, Brussels sprouts, bok choy, arugula) are also best eaten raw since they have the most powerful anticancer effects of all foods.

A high raw plant-based diet also tends to be very alkaline. What is alkaline and why is that so important? Our bodies should be 70 percent alkaline and 30 percent acid. The problem is that many of us are eating a highly acidic diet of processed meats, cheeses, breads, energy drinks, sodas, cigarettes, coffee, and alcohol. We are eating an extremely large amount of food with ingredients that have been chemically altered in a lab. Take a look at a food label—those words you can't pronounce? They're pronounced: acidic.

Our lives are also very acidic with all the pollution and stress we encounter daily. If we become too acidic, we create an environment in our bodies for illness and disease; we feel pain and we experience weight gain. When we become overly acidic, our bodies go into survival mode. To keep us alive our bodies will do a number of things:

1. Acids will store in our fat. This is one reason why we can cut calories, feed on "diet" foods, work out religiously, and still not lose weight. Our bodies are trying to save our lives by *holding onto fat*. Don't forget, "diet" foods are highly processed with chemicals, which means more acidity.

2. Acids will try to draw on our alkaline reserves by going to our teeth and bones for alkaline.

3. Acids will dehydrate you and make you thirsty. When I was at my most acidic, I experienced an unquenchable thirst. I drank a gallon of water during the day, and would keep a 32-ounce water bottle by my bedside at night. My body was trying to save my life by washing out the acids.

4. Many people in chronic pain are highly acidic. The excess acid aggravates pain. The only way to reduce the pain is to reduce the acid.

ACID FOODS

It's too bad that often the foods we like most make us most acidic. What are these foods?

Processed foods (foods with ingredients you can't pronounce)

Processed sugar, processed honey, and artificial sweeteners

Grains: (white) wheat, rice, pasta, flour, bread, etc.

Canned fruits and processed fruit juices

Bad fats: hydrogenated oils, corn oil, sunflower oil, margarine, and lard

Energy drinks, sodas, beer, wine, liquor, black tea, cigarettes

Peanuts

All animal products*: meat, fish, shellfish, eggs, butter, all dairy

---

* Note: Animal sources are very important for getting vitamin B12. Since they contain more acid than alkaline, animal products (if you do eat them) should be consumed in moderation. And always choose animals that have been treated humanely, fed organically, and raised free of antibiotics and hormones.

A WORD ON MODERATION

An exclusively raw diet is not for everyone—in fact, there are a few instances in which it is actually beneficial to incorporate cooked foods. Since many vitamins are water soluble, they are lost when cooking—except when steaming vegetables or making soups and stews where only a small portion of the nutrients are lost and many more nutrients are better able to be absorbed when moisturized. Also, in the case of soups and stews, we consume the liquid portion as well, where the nutrients remain. Unlike many raw foodists, I am not a purist. Ninety percent of my diet is raw, but occasionally, I incorporate soups, stews, and even salmon into my repertoire when I listen to my body's cravings. (See Chapter 5: Things Get Heated.)

ALKALINE FOODS

The majority of the foods we eat are highly acidic and can make us sick and tired. By eating raw alkaline foods and drinks, you can help your body maintain the ideal alkaline-acid balance. What are these foods?

All vegetables, especially raw green leafy vegetables

Fresh herbs and spices: parsley, basil, cilantro, cayenne, ginger

Sprouts

Sea vegetables and algaes

All fruits*, especially watermelon, avocado, cucumber, young coconuts

Grains: farro, quinoa, amaranth, buckwheat, and millet

Good fats: cold-pressed olive oil and unrefined coconut oil

Raw unprocessed sugars like raw honey and dates

---

* Note: Even though citrus fruits like lemons and limes are highly acidic before entering the body, once they are digested and assimilated, they are very alkaline.

▪ WHERE DO I GET MY PROTEIN? ▪

When we eat animal protein, our bodies have to use great reserves of energy to break down these proteins into amino acids. So I took the viewpoint that instead of eating animals, which my body would have to work hard to digest, I would skip the "middle man" and just eat the amino acids to give my body much-needed time to rest and "cleanse." Amino acids are found in all fruits, vegetables, nuts, seeds, and sprouts *before* you cook them.

After three years following a raw vegan diet and enjoying my time of "cleansing," I started to feel my health decline. My body was craving something. What? With just a little investigating I found exactly what fit the bill. I began to add a raw egg to my Happy Shake (page 3) each morning. I immediately felt improvement. A few months later I added some seared fish to my diet a couple of times a week and really felt satiated. Some people who follow strictly raw vegan diets for extended periods of time can start to feel deficiencies. For me, the problem seemed to be a lack of vitamin B12—and eggs and fish are great sources of B12.

I never adopted this diet with the intention of becoming a vegan. So my deci-

CAN I STOP OBSESSING ABOUT CALORIES?

Yes! This is my first gift to you: Instead of obsessing about calories and restriction, our goal is to let go of processed foods. Our bodies thrive on raw unprocessed foods. This more alkaline diet of real food will slowly allow us to shed those extra pounds, or at least maintain a healthy weight for our bodies.

sion to add eggs and fish to my diet was an easy one. My goal has always been to eat in a way that gives me a feeling of vibrancy, health, and happiness. I also prefer getting my vitamin B12 from a food source rather than a supplement. This does not mean you can't be a successful vegan. You just have to be vigilant with regards to testing your blood and supplementing your diet to ensure optimal nutrition.

If you choose to eat from an animal source, make sure the animals have been treated humanely and with respect. Look for animals that are not given steroids, hormones, or antibiotics. Find eggs that are organic and cage free. We may not always have access to the freshest ingredients or the healthiest food in every situation, but being mindful of our nutritional intake and making the best possible choices from the options we have is an attainable goal—one that I share with each of the families I cook with, and that is my hope for you in making the change to a mostly raw food diet.

▪ TAKE ME TO A STEAKHOUSE ▪

"How do you eat out?"

This is a question I hear quite often and that is a very easy question to answer. First and foremost is *attitude*. When I join friends for an evening out, I go with the purpose of enjoying their company, not with eating the perfect raw meal. As I always say, people first and then food.

Keep in mind that *Eat Raw, Not Cooked* is not about a 100 percent raw or vegan philosophy. There is no food religion to join or titles to adopt. My purpose is to introduce you to the tastiest ways of adding more wholesome raw foods into your diet, not to become a "raw foodist," which to me sounds close to "raw nudist." You can now enjoy, guilt-free, some steamed broccoli or roasted Brussels sprouts on that green salad you just ordered. Bon appetit!

Believe it or not, my favorite restaurants are steakhouses. A steakhouse always provides a nice big fluffy salad. I ask for some olive oil and lemon and set about enjoying my greens while enjoying my friends' company. Sometimes I get a really amazing salad. Sometimes it's kinda wimpy. But I always try to keep in mind that

RAW FOODIES CAN BE FATTIES, TOO

The key to good health is balance and moderation in everything. This means don't just live on desserts, even raw desserts. You gotta eat your greens (they are uber alkalizing)! My personal rule of thumb: Eat fresh real food only when you are hungry, work hard, stay active, keep family and friends close, enjoy life, laugh!

I am there for the people I am with, not for the best salad in town. I also happen to love fish and can always find a nice piece of fish to accompany my salad.

Dining out is simply about making better choices. You just have to learn to scan the menu for greens and fresh vegetables. The sides and salads are perfect places to start. Pretty soon your eyes will automatically key into these healthier options. Don't be afraid to ask for a substitute. I always recommend substituting the nutritionally poor starchy white carbohydrates loaded with butter for more greens. I have a favorite sports bar in Chicago called Mother Hubbard's, located on Hubbard Street. I order up their amazing supersize bowl of guacamole and a side of steamed broccoli instead of the chips—I call it, "Broccomole"!

Before a recent flight from San Francisco to New York, with little time to prepare, I made a quick stop at a local market to scan the aisles for something to pack in my carry-on. I wound up with some prewashed romaine leaves, two avocados, and one California sweet orange. Armed with my little wooden travel utensils, I sliced up my avocado and folded it into the romaine leaves for some "Avocado Roll Ups"—a creation born of desperation that made for a rich and satisfying snack to get me through a day of travel.

▪ NOURISH YOUR KIDS ▪
. . . WITHOUT THEM KNOWING*

The number one reason families invite me into their homes is to learn about healthier food choices for their kids. Before I even set foot in a family's home, I learn about the kids first. What are their ages? What are their go-to snacks? Do they like fruits or vegetables? What are their favorite flavors and family dinners? Do they like dessert?

---

* this technique works on reluctant spouses as well . . . .

Today, more and more kids have food allergies to some level or degree. This is very common in the homes I visit. My goal here is to get the whole family involved in food preparation, while bringing yummy solutions and *fun* into the kitchen.

I begin by telling the parents to keep their kids' current favorite foods in the house as an option for the dinner table, even if this includes chicken fingers or macaroni and cheese. Change in diet is hard enough for adults and much harder for children. Be gentle with your kids and make the kitchen a safe and loving place with choices they themselves can make.

Avoid hovering over their plates like a helicopter. How do *you* feel when others are overly focused on your plate? The more you push a new food or diet on them, the more resistance you will receive. Keep in mind, even if unintentionally, you are the one who led them down the addictive path of high-sugared juices, boxed cereals, and processed foods. Not all is lost though, so don't be hard on yourself! You were doing the best you knew with the knowledge you had. My best advice is to lead by example and *have fun* with food.

▪ STUFF FOR MAKING STUFF: ▪ YOUR TOOLS AND STAPLES

Let's start with a quick introduction to my favorite kitchen tools, as well as a few ingredients that may be new to you. You will be able to find most things at your local health food markets; if the more obscure ingredients prove hard to find, they are just a mouse click away from your kitchen. This is why I love Google!

TOOLS

My favorite tool, your own two hands: These are quite possibly the most powerful and overlooked tools ever! I use my hands for everything. They are perfect for spreading mixtures evenly when making breads or crackers. I find my hands especially useful for plating a beautifully presented dish.

Bamboo utensils: I love my little wooden travel utensils by To-Go Wear (www .togowear.com). I use them when traveling, but I also really love eating my Happy Shake (page 3) with a wooden spoon at home. I find I am a little protective of my wooden spoons. I also enjoy a wood cutting board, plates, and salad bowls. What a nice organic way to eat.

Ceramic knife: You are going to be doing a lot of cutting and chopping. A good knife is key. I love my ceramic knives. I never have to sharpen them. (Kyocera, a Japanese company, makes great knives that come in some pretty cool colors.)

Dehydrator: I make crackers, breads, snacks, and cookies in a food dehydrator at 115°F. The dehydrator I recommend is the Excalibur five-tray or nine-tray model. You will also need to order nonstick dehydrator sheets for making breads and crackers.

Food processor: The food processor has interchangeable blades, used for shredding, blending, chopping, or slicing. I have used some very expensive brands and I have also had success with very inexpensive ones. I do prefer a processor with a larger container. Choose what works best for your budget.

Immersion blender: An immersion blender is basically a stick with blender blades at the end of it, used for blending soups and sauces. You can use it right in the pot on the stove—this saves time and is so convenient, especially for large amounts of soup.

Julienne peeler: I keep one of these at home in my own kitchen, and one stays in my suitcase. I love it soooooo much! A julienne peeler is a hand-held kitchen utensil that cuts vegetables into thin, even strips, in a style known as a julienne cut. These julienne strips dress up many dishes and serves as a raw "noodle" in my Asian and Italian dishes. You get what you pay for with this product. Splurge on the best. A really nice one will run you $15 to $20.

Lemon squeezer: Another tool I never leave home without; every home should have one! (The Amco aluminum squeezer is my favorite; it's easy to use and comes in a fun citrus color.)

Mason jars: Wide-mouth Mason jars (32 ounces) are the BEST—they are cheap, too. I use them for storing nuts, seeds, superfoods, sauces, dressings, and leftover soups. I love drinking out of them. These 32-ounce jars let me know I am drinking my daily intake of water.

Nut milk bag (or filtering bag): This is a nylon bag great for making nut milks, seed milks, and juices. Order online from Vermont Fiddle Heads (www.vt-fiddle.com).

Spiralizer: For a nice bowl of angel hair "pasta," use the Spiralizer. You just secure your zucchini onto a prong, turn a handle, and thin noodles form. This little contraption took me a bit of practice and a YouTube instructional video to get it right, but once I got going, I took off like a noodle pro!

Turning slicer: This type of slicer is perfect for making thick twisty "noodles" for Mac & Cheeze (page 92). The overall best one on the market (which you can find online) is World Cuisine Tri-Blade Plastic Vegetable Slicer. I love how quickly I can zip right through a squash, creating a big bowl of "noodles." Clean up is easy and the price of this slicer is around $30. These noodles bring a lot of fun to the dinner table.

Vitamix: Where do I start? This is a miracle machine! With a hefty price tag of $500, it is worth every penny. Don't be duped into opting for anything less. If you can't afford the Vitamix, make due with your basic blender ($30) and save up your pennies for the Vitamix. Trust me. The Vitamix is a great and durable machine and will likely save you time and money in the end.

The Vitamix is a 2.5-horsepower high-speed blender that is famous for capabilities beyond what you would expect from any other blender. It comes with a "tamper/accelerator" (that's what they call it); this is sort of like a rubber plunger thingy used for pushing down and processing thick, dense ingredients that would bring all other blenders to a halt. The Vitamix also comes with (for an extra price) a dry-grain container that is excellent for grinding nuts, seeds, and grains into flours. I don't know how I ever lived without this attachment. (No, I don't get any commission checks for promoting the Vitamix. I just love this machine!)

STAPLES

Agave, raw: A low-glycemic liquid sweetener. I treat raw agave like any other sweetener, as a treat.

Almond butter: What a great butter for sauces and spreads. Look for the raw unroasted butter.

Apple cider vinegar: This is my vinegar of choice. Raw apple cider vinegar is very alkaline-forming in the body and a great digestive aid.

Cacao nibs and powder: Yes! Raw unprocessed chocolate is good for you! It is the #1 weight loss food, the #1 antioxidant food—full of LOVE chemicals. Raw chocolate is BLISS!

Cacao paste: When preparing raw chocolate candies, many people will melt together raw cacao butter and raw cacao powder. I find cacao paste so much easier to work with; it's already blended, eliminating that middle step. Buy cacao paste online from www.vt-fiddle.com.

Carob: A great chocolate substitute for those sensitive to chocolate. Look for the unroasted fresh ground carob.

Chia seeds: These are tiny, supernutritious, gelatinous seeds, great in puddings and shakes.

Coconut, shredded: Look for organic, unsweetened, dried coconut in most health food stores.

Coconut milk, canned: I use canned coconut milk in recipes for convenience. Cracking open coconuts can be tricky, expensive, and disappointing . . . unless of course you live in the tropics and have a machete. My brand of choice is a PBA-free organic coconut milk by Native Forest.

Coconut oil (unrefined): This oil actually helps you lose weight! This is because of the presence of medium-chain saturated fatty acids present in coconut products. It is also a great beauty aid for hair and skin. For the most health benefits, choose "unrefined" coconut oil. Coconut oil is the only oil that does not turn toxic when heated. When cooking, you can cook with "refined" coconut oil.

Coconut palm sugar: Coconut palm sugar is a completely natural, unrefined sugar coming from the flowers growing high on top of coconut trees. This sugar is low-glycemic (meaning no "sugar crash") and rich in key phytonutrients, vitamins, and minerals, including potassium, iron, zinc, vitamins B1, B2, B3, and B6.

Dates: Medjool dates have been called the "king of dates." They are exceptionally sweet and a very good source of fiber. These dates are my first choice when making desserts. Be sure to take out the pits. Most dates are not as juicy as the Medjool date. If choosing another kind of date, you may need more than the recipe calls for. If your dates are too dry, you may need to add a tiny bit of water to your recipe.

Dulse: Rich in trace minerals from the sea, this sea vegetable is a welcome accompaniment or garnish to salads, or can simply be enjoyed as a healthy snack.

Farro: High in fiber, vitamin B, and protein, farro is an ancient grain that has been long loved in Italy for it's delicious nutty flavor and chewy texture. It has a low gluten content and can be tolerated by most of those with wheat allergies.

Fermented Gingered Carrots: These colorful carrots from Real Pickles (www.realpickles .com) have a wonderful gingery zing—great on any salad dish or rolled into spring rolls—and are made with 100 percent organic ingredients: carrots, ginger, filtered water, unrefined sea salt.

Hemp seeds: Hemp seeds are omega-rich and full of protein. Enjoy sprinkled into salads and smoothies.

Honey, raw: Honey in its raw and organic state is rich in minerals, antioxidants, probiotics, and enzymes. It's a very healing and digestible sugar to our bodies.

Kalamata olives: Kalamata olives are popular Greek black olives available in most large supermarkets. They are salty and very flavorful—definitely my first choice in an olive.

Lecithin: Lecithin is an emulsifier, full of B vitamins and used in desserts for binding liquids with oils. Since lecithin is a soy product, make sure you choose one that is a non-GMO and organic.

Maca: Maca is a hearty little root grown on the mountains of Peru that is great for men and women's sexual health. Perfect for easing symptoms of menopause and enhancing sexual libido, maca greatly affects stamina, endurance, mental clarity, and depression. As an adaptogen, maca will help us adapt to the stressful situations life sometimes hands us.

Maple syrup, Grade B: Grade B maple syrup is the most minimally processed of the maple syrups, making it more nutrient-dense. Whatever you do, for heaven's sake, get off those fake pancake syrups!

Millet: Although millet is often associated with what people put in their bird feeders, it's not just for the birdies. Millet is packed full of nutrients and fiber. It's a heart-healthy grain.

Nori: Nori is another sea vegetable rich in nutrition. Sea vegetables improve digestion, help regulate metabolism, glandular and hormonal flows, and can calm our nervous systems. Be sure to purchase untoasted nori.

Nutritional yeast flakes: These are dried flakes, full of B vitamins and a cheesy flavor. Find them in bulk at your local health food store.

Nuts (cashews, almonds, pecans, walnuts, macadamia nuts, pine nuts): Always look for raw and organic nuts. There are many online suppliers to choose from if your local market does not carry them.

Olive oil: Look for "First Cold Pressed" olive oil in your markets.

Pickle relish (raw): Bubbies Pure Kosher Dill Relish is made with no sugar, no vinegar or preservatives—we can finally enjoy a healthy pickle relish! It is great in tartar sauce or served on a "burger."

Sauerkraut (raw): Raw kraut is a highly nutritious, low-fat, low-calorie food. Raw kraut contains lactic acid bacteria, digestive enzymes, and vitamin C. Raw kraut is a natural probiotic, excellent for our digestive systems! Always choose raw unpasteurized kraut in order to maintain all the nutritional benefits.

Sea salt: Typical table salt found in markets has been flash-dried at extremely high temperatures and chemically bleached. Choose a nice pink or grey sea salt loaded with minerals.

Seeds (sunflower, sesame, golden flax): Always look for raw and organic seeds. There are many online suppliers to choose from if your local market does not carry them.

Teeccino: Made from carob, barley, chicory, dates, and almonds, Teeccino is a great coffee alternative. Brew it just like coffee, add a little raw cacao, almond milk, and coconut palm sugar to taste for a super cafe mocha.

EAT YOUR CHOCOLATE (CACAO) RAW!

A POWERFUL ANTIOXIDANT: By weight, raw cacao has more antioxidants than red wine, green tea, acai, pomegranates, and blueberries combined. Antioxidants protect us from age-related illnesses.

FOR WEIGHT MANAGEMENT: Phenylethylamine (PEA) is a chemical produced in our body when we fall in love. It increases focus, alertness, and serves as a natural appetite suppressant. We can produce this chemical at will by eating raw cacao.

THE HAPPY FOOD: Anandamide is a "bliss" chemical found in raw cacao, and tryptophan is an amazing mood-enhancing amino acid found in raw cacao.

Vanilla: I use pure organic vanilla extract, which can be found in most supermarkets and health food stores. When shopping, watch out for any extracts labeled "imitation vanilla" or "vanilla flavoring"—this is not vanilla.

Vitamineral Green: Vitamineral Green is a 100 percent green-focused superfood by HealthForce Nutritionals. Greens are the most healing foods on the planet and the single most important addition to your diet, especially in the RAW! Vitamineral Green is not a supplement; it is food. Add it to your morning smoothies. (Order online at healthforce.com.)

WHAT IS THE BEST JUICER?

With the help of the right juicer, you can have freshly pressed juice right at home, every day. There are two types of juicers: centrifugal and cold-pressed. Although both machines provide you with fresh juice, how they operate and the juice they provide is very different.

Centrifugal juicers are the most common juicers on the market. They are quick and easy to use. They clean up fast. However, the centrifugal force of the blade heats up and oxidizes the juice. This gives you a juice that has fewer nutrients than a pressed juice. If you do use this juicer, be sure to drink your juice immediately after juicing.

Cold-press juicers press the vegetables. This produces a richer juice. This juice can actually be bottled and stored in your refrigerator for 2 to 3 days because the cold press does not oxidize the vegetables. For maximum healing benefits, you want a cold-press or masticating juicer. These juicers tend to be more expensive, slower juicing, and more time-consuming to clean than the centrifugal juicer.

In the end, the best juicer for you is the juicer you will actually use. And if you are short on time and/or patience, juice bars are the best! There is no juicer to clean, and you can get your juice on the run.

eat
raw,
not
cooked

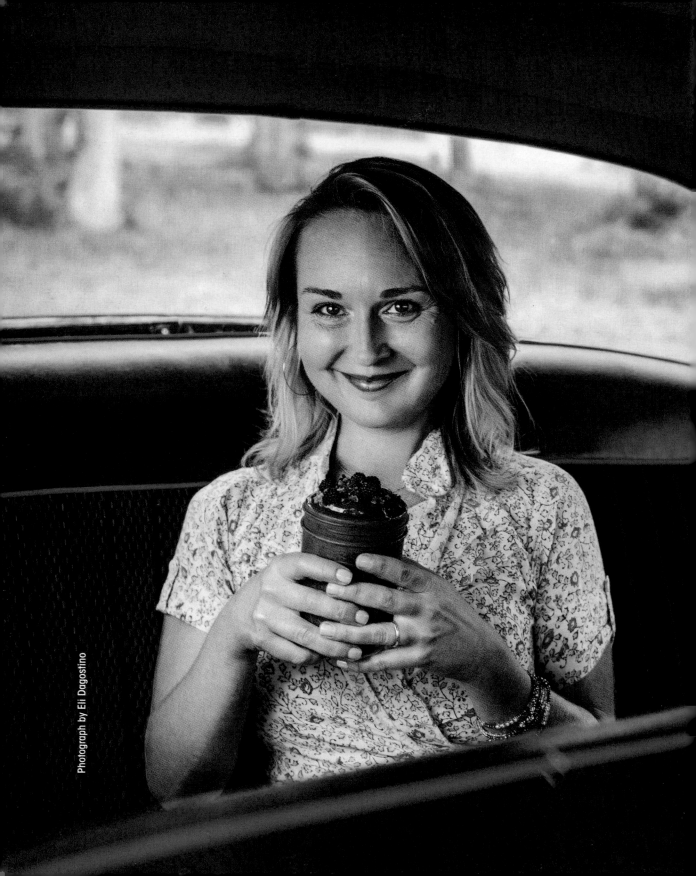

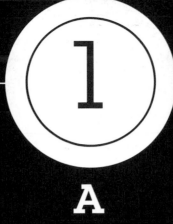

A Salad in Disguise . . .

When I first began the raw food diet, I discovered that all these "Raw Foodies" were drinking something called green smoothies. They would take fruits and a lot of green leaves, throw them into a blender, blend, and drink. Next thing I knew, I was throwing green leaves and fruits into my little blender. It was definitely *green*—it tasted like my dad's lawn clippings to me.

Why a green smoothie? Greens are rich in nutrients, minerals, antioxidants, and enzymes, and when blended into a green smoothie, these greens are very easily digested. Green smoothies aid in cleansing and healing the body, they boost your immune system, and because they are rich in nutrients, you will feel less hungry and more satisfied, so you can lose excess weight, have fewer cravings, and feel healthier and happier!

My first goal was to take this green glass of lawn clippings and turn it into something I would be happy to enjoy myself and even happier to share with others. The result? The Happy Shake (page 3), a salad disguised as a soft serve ice cream that you eat with a spoon. Soft-serve ice cream has always been my favorite dessert and now I get to eat it for breakfast every morning. My wildest dreams have come true!

Before getting started, let's talk again about my favorite kitchen tool for making the perfect Happy Shake: the Vitamix. Trust me, it will make all your time in the kitchen much more pleasurable. However, if you cannot afford one, you can still make the Happy Shake in the cheapest of little blenders. You will just need to exercise a bit more patience, but it can be done. The Vitamix comes with a handy plunger for pushing down the fruit. If you are working with a traditional blender, use a carrot as your plunger and slowly add your fruits in while blending.

1

Photograph by Eli Dagostino

WENDY'S LARGE ORIGINAL CHOCOLATE FROSTY™ *

One of the most popular drive-through soft serve ice creams has always been the Wendy's Chocolate Frosty. I have definitely had my share! How do they make it so thick? Mostly with a barrage of thickening agents such as guar gum, cellulose gum, and carrageenan!

Ingredients: Milk, Sugar, Corn Syrup, Cream, Whey, Nonfat Milk, Cocoa (processed with alkali), **Guar Gum**, Mono and Diglycerides, **Cellulose Gum, Carrageenan**, Calcium Sulfate, Disodium Phosphate, Artificial Flavor, Vitamin A Palmitate.

Per serving: 590 calories, 15g fat, 97g carbohydrates, 81g sugar, 17g protein

* Ingredients and nutrition information for this and other restaurant or packaged products referenced in this book were accessed from the companies' websites in 2013. Nutrition and ingredients lists can change. For the most up-to-date information, please visit the applicable company or product website.

THE HAPPY SHAKE

Though this creamy blend tastes like a delicious dessert, it's chock-full of spinach, berries, and super happy foods, like raw chocolate and maca. The Happy Shake is a meal replacement. It's a key place to start when trying to lose excess weight, increase energy levels, and get healthier—and happier! Before you get started, keep in mind the Happy Shake is more about technique than anything else. You can take these same ingredients, throw them into a blender, and get a glass full of lawn clippings. So follow the directions closely.

½ cup water

3 to 4 cups spinach

1 tablespoon coconut oil or 1 organic egg

1 tablespoon raw maca powder

2 tablespoons raw cacao powder

1 cup frozen blueberries

¾ cup frozen cherries

¼ cup frozen banana, sliced in small pieces before freezing

Optional: a little raw honey for those who like extra sweetness

Optional: 3 ice cubes or a small handful of ice for those hot humid days

Toppings: Raw cacao nibs, goji berries, shredded coconut, or fresh local bee pollen

1. The Base: In your Vitamix or blender start with the water.

2. The Greens: Here is your salad! Use a mild tasting green like spinach. Kale is way too bitter and *not* happy.

3. A Good Fat: Add the coconut oil or egg. Good fat won't make you fat, and is essential for metabolizing the greens and keeping you feeling satisfied longer. Be sure to add the fat after the greens, or it will get stuck on the bottom! Do not be tempted to leave out the fat. If you are adding a raw egg, use less water.

4. The HAPPY Parts: Add the maca powder and cacao powder.

5. Blend all of these ingredients until they yield 1 cup of green sludge. (Do not add the fruit until *after* making the sludge—this is very important for getting the right consistency.) Add the 2 cups frozen fruit. (You can use any combination of blueberries, blackberries, cherries, strawberries, raspberries, and bananas. My personal favorite combination is blueberry/cherry. Find your favorite combo!) If you are using a tradi-

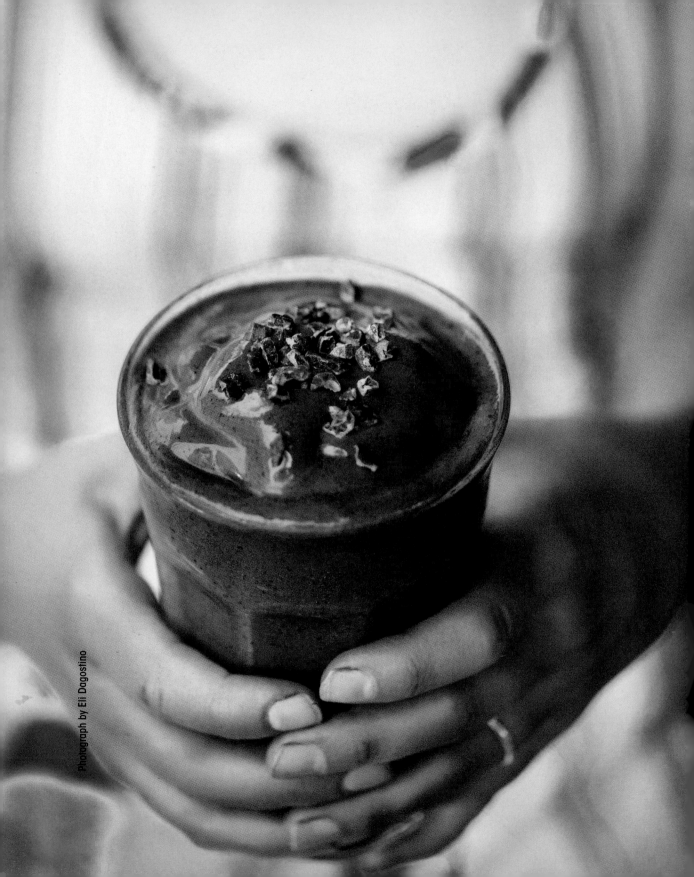

tional blender, a carrot will be helpful for pushing your frozen fruit down the sides of the blender. This will give you a more efficient blend. The blending time is short to get a thick ice cream–like consistency. Do not overblend; overblending will yield more of a shakelike drink instead of the desired soft-serve ice cream texture. You'll get the hang of it with practice.

6. The Toppings: Now it's time to decorate your Happy Shake. I like to add some raw cacao nibs. You can also top with goji berries, shredded coconut, or fresh local bee pollen.

1 large serving: 344 calories, 14.9g fat, 54.9g carbohydrates, 32g sugar, 5.8g protein

SERVES 1

A NOTE ON COLOR . . .

The blueberries are important for getting the chocolatey brown color, so use plenty of blues! The best are frozen wild blueberries.

GREEN sludge + BLUEberries = Chocolate BROWN!

VARIATION: THE MILDLY AMUSED

When it comes to young children and some sensitive adults, I recommend the Mildly Amused—it has everything you get in the Happy Shake, minus the maca or cacao. While these foods are not harmful for most, they are foods with medicinal benefits. Again, research new foods when adding them to your family's diets. A great alternative to those sensitive to cacao is raw carob powder. Raw carob is a great food for promoting healthy digestion.

A NOTE ON SUPERFOODS . . .

Superfoods like maca, cacao, and bee pollen are very powerful. Do your own research on these amazing superfoods. Just because they work great for me does not mean they will work for you. Start in small doses and listen to your body. Superfoods can be ordered online or may also be located at your local health food stores.

A SALAD IN DISGUISE . . .

ENERGY DRINKS

Can energy drinks really send you to the hospital or be fatal? It's possible. These products have become incredibly popular with teens and college students. Red Bull, Monster, 5-Hour Energy, Jolt, and Rockstar may be marketed as sexy or cool, but can prove to be deadly. Since these beverages are sold as "drinks," the FDA does not require them to state the amount of caffeine on their product. The problem is, there are people who are more sensitive to these high doses of caffeine than others. Risks with ingesting so much caffeine include disturbed sleep, which translates to less focus during the day and/or heart palpitations. These palpitations can drastically increase the risk of heart problems, including heart attacks.

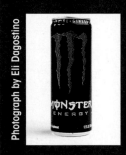

Photograph by Eli Dagostino

An energy drink seems like a quick and easy fix. For real energy, lets make green juice the new cool!

Ingredients: Carbonated Water, Sucrose, Glucose, Citric Acid, Natural Flavors, Taurine, Sodium Citrate, Color Added, Panax Ginseng, Root Extract, L-Carnitine, Caffeine, Sorbic Acid, Benzoic Acid, Niacinamide, Sodium Chloride, Glucuronolactone, Inositol, Hydrochloride, Sucralose, Riboflavin, Maltodextrin, Cyanocobalamin.

THE REPLENISHER

Why juice? When we juice our vegetables, we get a highly concentrated drink of nutrients that are able to enter our bloodstream quickly. Start by drinking 16 to 24 ounces of a freshly pressed green juice a day, and watch your energy increase and your skin glow within a week!

2 cucumbers	1 kiwifruit, peeled
3 celery stalks	1 lime, peeled
2 green apples, cored	1 thumb-size piece of fresh ginger, peeled
1 handful of parsley	*Optional*: 1 slice jalapeño pepper
4–5 lacinato kale leaves	(a great addition!)

Juice your vegetables according to your specific juicer's directions and drink your salad!

SERVES 2

Note: Organic is always the best choice for so many reasons. Organic produce is free from pesticides, herbicides, fungicides, insecticides, and gases used for ripening. Organic animal products lessen your exposure to antibiotics, synthetic hormones, and drugs. All of the above are potentially cancer causing. Choosing organic also means you are supporting family farmers who can create for themselves a livelihood. Choosing organics is the domestic version of fair trade. I like fair! Organics are higher in nutrients than nonorganics. To top it off, organics simply taste better!

Sadly today, with growing economic stresses on our families, it has become a privilege to eat food that has not been sprayed with chemicals. Don't let organic vs. nonorganic keep you from adding more raw foods to your diet. Before I knew anything about "organic food," I found healing on a raw nonorganic diet. This says a lot for the power of RAW foods!

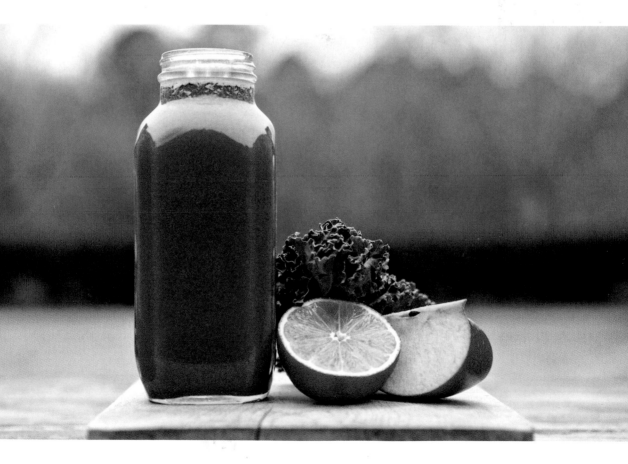

A SALAD IN DISGUISE . . .

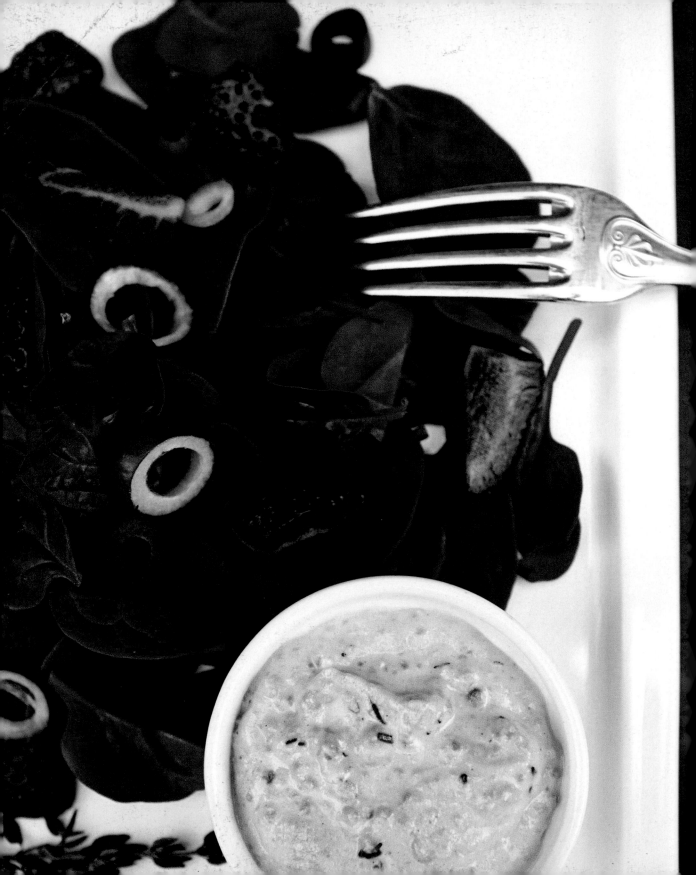

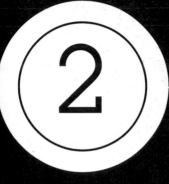

Dress Up Your Greens

DRESSINGS, DIPS, and SAUCES

Home on the Range Dressing

"Chips" & Dip

Better Than Ketchup & "Fries"

Creamy Honey Mustard Dressing

Not Peanut Sauce

Basic White Sauce . . . The Perfect Cream Cheeze

The Champion Caesar Salad Dressing

Honey's Dijon Vinaigrette

Susie's Spicy Curry Sauce

Honey Girl's Strawberry Vinaigrette

Not-Cho-Cheeze Sauce

Tyrannosaurus Red Sauce

Super Simple Marinade

Not Blue Cheese Dressing

Wicked Cole Slaw Dressing

Dips and sauces are going to turn your salad fixins' into some really spectacular and creative meals and snacks. We all know we should eat our vegetables. Simply put, vegetables are the highest quality food on the planet. Rich in nutrients and fiber, they should be the centerpiece of our dinner plates. Let's make good use of this abundant variety of beautiful gifts! The first step in enjoying your vegetables is a good foundation.

▪ The Foundation: A Good Dressing ▪

Put down the bottle! Making your own dressings can be simple, fun, creative, and oh so much healthier. If you take a peek at the ingredients on any store-bought bottled dressings, you'd better have a dictionary handy. I say: If you can't pronounce it, don't eat it.

The dressing recipes here will serve as a guideline for you. I have found that when making recipes for families, everyone has their own preferences and tastes. I will share with you the most popular versions. If something doesn't work for you, tweak it and create your own dressings, dips, and sauces. Since these recipes yield quite a bit of sauce, I like to use the dressings as a base for a whole new creation the next day or within the week.

▪ Harvest Your Greens ▪

Green leaves are at the top of my vegetable chain. Always have a supply of washed greens on hand—cleaning and cutting them ahead of time will streamline your preparation. No one wants to walk in the door hungry and have to rummage through a fridge full of unprepared vegetables. I keep a salad spinner in my refrigerator. This is a wonderful tool for cleaning and keeping your greens fresh. I always have a variety of fresh clean greens waiting to be enjoyed.

I am very careful not to waste one precious little vegetable that makes its way into my kitchen. So I don't overbuy produce or overprepare. I just make a regular routine of stopping by my local farmers' market or local grocer a couple of times a week. I promise this is an investment that will pay off, not only in your health, but in your wallet as well.

■ Before We Get Started, ■
a Word on Soaking Your Nuts . . .

Many of these recipes are nut free, but the creamier dressings will use nuts. If you are using a traditional little blender, I suggest soaking your nuts first. Yes, I said it, "Soak your nuts, folks." You can soak them at room temperature for a couple of hours or overnight in your refrigerator. This will make blending them into a creamy sauce so much easier. In the recipes, I will not call for you to soak your nuts. I will assume you have a high-speed blender and are so busy that you are happy to skip this step.

There is also another good reason to soak your nuts. When you soak them, you release enzyme inhibitors, which make them easier to digest. Always rinse your nuts after you soak them because you don't want to eat those little acidic inhibitors that are released. Use or dehydrate soaked nuts right away to ensure that they don't get moldy. No one wants moldy nuts.

CASHEWS FOR WEIGHT MANAGEMENT?

Yes! Even though cashew nuts have a high fat content, these fats are considered "good fats." Cashew nuts have a high energy density, along with being high in fiber, which make them great for weight management when eaten in moderation. The creamy fattiness in a raw cashew is perfect for re-creating recipes that typically call for butter or dairy, commonly known allergens.

Note: These amazing dressings, dips, and sauces will be thicker or thinner depending on how much water you add to them; when stored in the refrigerator, they will thicken up—you may need to add more water after storing. Most of these dressings store well for at least ten days because they are all dairy-free. Have fun "Dressing Up Your Greens"!

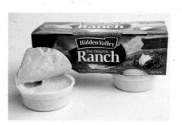

2

HIDDEN VALLEY RANCH DRESSING

What's in this most popular Midwestern condiment? Reading through the list below, we start off fairly positive and quickly decline. If your family frequents restaurants or eats processed foods, you are more than likely indulging in one of the scariest ingredients out there, MSG (monosodium glutamate).

Dr. Russell Blaylock, a board-certified neurosurgeon and author of *Excitotoxins: The Taste That Kills*, explains that MSG is an excitotoxin, which means it overexcites your cells to the point of damage or death, causing brain damage to varying degrees and potentially even triggering or worsening learning disabilities, Alzheimer's disease, Parkinson's disease, Lou Gehrig's disease, and more.

Ingredients: Vegetable Oil, Water, Egg Yolk, Sugar, Salt, Cultured Nonfat Buttermilk, Natural Flavors, Spices, Dried Garlic, Dried Onion, Vinegar, Phosphoric Acid, Xanthan Gum, Modified Food Starch, **Monosodium Glutamate,** Artificial Flavors, Disodium Phosphate, Sorbic Acid, Calcium Disodium EDTA, Disodium Inosinate, Disodium Guanylate.

HOME ON THE RANGE DRESSING

This is my version of America's favorite dressing—ranch!

2 cups raw cashews

1 cup olive oil

½ cup fresh lemon juice

1¼ cups water
(or to taste for desired consistency)

¼ cup apple cider vinegar

2 tablespoons raw agave nectar or raw honey

⅓ cup chopped red onion

3 small garlic cloves

1½ teaspoons sea salt

1 teaspoon dried basil

1 teaspoon dried dill

In a high-speed blender, combine the cashews, oil, lemon juice, water, vinegar, agave, onion, garlic, and salt and blend until creamy. Add the basil and dill and quick-blend, until you see little flecks of green. This creates added flavor for the *eyes*. Do not overblend. Serve immediately as a dressing or dip. This dressing thickens once chilled. Add additional water to thin it out.

MAKES 35 OUNCES

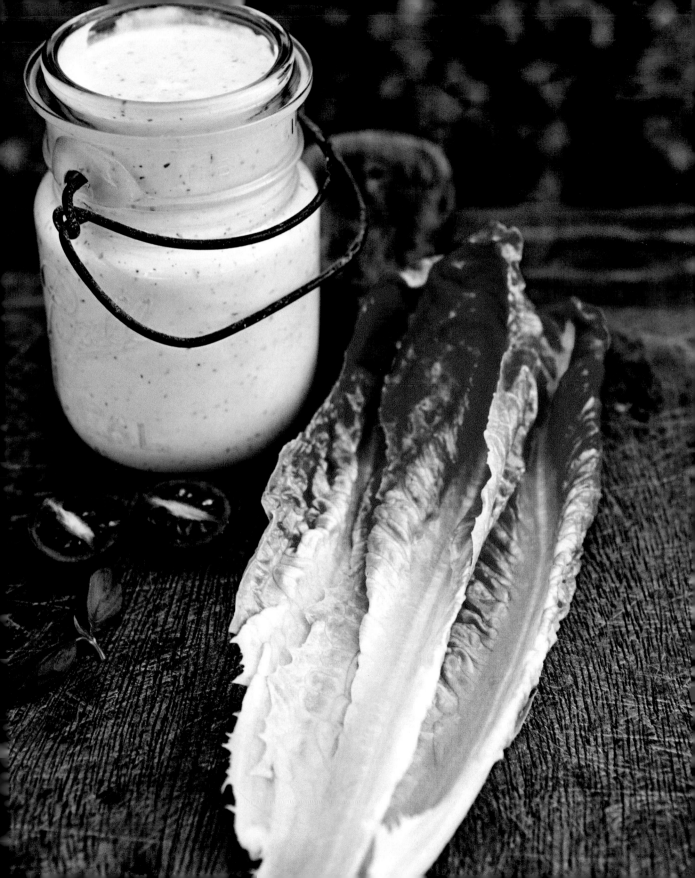

3

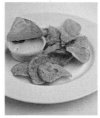

LAY'S® CLASSIC POTATO CHIP

Ingredients: Potatoes, Vegetable Oil (Sunflower, Corn, and/or Canola Oil), and Salt. No Preservatives.

Wow! Sounds pretty innocent, right? Wrong. Vegetable oils like canola oil, soybean oil, corn oil, sunflower oil, safflower oil, and margarine are all extracted using a chemical process developed in the early 1900s. Before then, these oils were practically nonexistent; now they are some of the most chemically altered foods on store shelves today. Yet they keep getting promoted as healthy—and we keep getting heart disease.

MEET YOUR "CHIP"!

1. Heart-healthy vitamin C: Move over, oranges. One serving of romaine lettuce contains 40% of your recommended daily needs of vitamin C. Interestingly, vitamin C prevents cholesterol from sticking to the walls of your blood vessels. Thus, if you have a strong family history of heart disease, you should include a couple of servings of romaine lettuce in your daily diet to keep your heart healthy.

2. Mineral-rich: We may assume the dark leafy greens like kale are superior, but don't let romaine's light color fool you. One head contains copper (33% RDA), magnesium (22% RDA), manganese (42% RDA), phosphorus (27% RDA), potassium (33% RDA), selenium (5% RDA), and zinc (13% RDA), not to mention calcium (see below) and iron (see below).

3. Calcium-rich: One head of romaine has 206mg of calcium (about 21% RDA).

4. Protein: You read right! Romaine lettuce is a complete protein, having all 18 essential amino acids. A head, 7.7g of protein, has 17% of the RDA.

5. Omega-3s: One head of romaine lettuce contains 44% RDA of omega-3 essential fats.

6. Iron-rich. One head of romaine contains 6mg of iron.

7. Low levels of oxalic acid: If you have problems with calcium oxalate kidney stones, romaine lettuce might be your leaf of choice, since it is very low in oxalic acid.

8. Hydration: One head of romaine provides about 20 ounces of water.

9. Rich source of vitamins A (as beta-carotene) and K: Romaine is super-rich in beta-carotene with 1,817% RDA per head and has 535% RDA of vitamin K.

10. Rich in B vitamins: Here are the percentages of the RDA for the B vitamins in romaine. Thiamine (B1), 38%; Riboflavin (B2), 32%; Niacin (B3), 12%; Pantothenic Acid (B5), 18%; Pyridoxine (B6), 36%; Folate (B9), 213%.

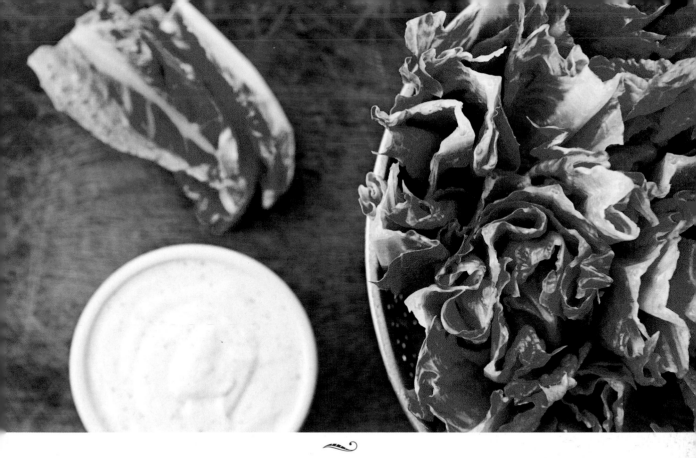

"CHIPS" & DIP

At almost every party I have ever been to, some sort of chips and dip are inevitably served. There is a comfort in dipping—it makes food fun. I am always encouraging my families to eat two salads a day. This means 8 cups of "fluffy" greens per day. Not all of us want to sit down to a salad twice a day, every day. So, I created the CHIP!

1 three-pack bag of crispy organic
hearts of romaine

Home on the Range Dressing (page 12)

Wash and cut your heads of romaine crosswise into thirds. This will give you 3-inch romaine chips, perfect for dipping. Display your chips in a large bowl, set out your dressing, and watch your guests enjoy a fun salad in disguise as their favorite comfort food.

YIELD: 3 SERVINGS

DRESS UP YOUR GREENS

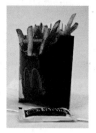

4

McDONALD'S MEDIUM FRENCH FRIES & KETCHUP

What's in a McDonald's French fry?

Ingredients: Potatoes, Partially Hydrogenated Soybean Oil, Natural Flavor (Beef, Wheat, and Dairy Sources), Dextrose, Sodium Acid Pyrophosphate. Cooked in partially hydrogenated vegetable oils.

What's in McDonald's ketchup?

Ingredients: Tomato Concentrate from Tomatoes, Distilled Vinegar, High Fructose Corn Syrup, Water, Salt, Natural Flavors.

Not all sweeteners are created equal when it comes to weight gain. A Princeton University research team discovers: Rats with access to high fructose corn syrup gained significantly more weight than those with access to table sugar, even when their overall caloric intake was the same.

~∼⊃

BETTER THAN KETCHUP & "FRIES"

Many Americans eat foods based on their potential to be dipped in ketchup. If you are one of those Americans, this recipe is for you! Try serving this alongside The Perfect Picnic Burger (page 90). The ketchup also makes a great pizza sauce on the Raw Pizzas (page 81).

KETCHUP
1 cup chopped tomatoes (about 1½ medium)
1 cup oil-packed sun-dried tomatoes, drained
¼ cup raw agave nectar
3 tablespoons apple cider vinegar

1 tablespoon tamari
1 small garlic clove
Optional: 1 tablespoon water

"FRIES"
Yellow squash or jicama

1. For the ketchup: In a blender, combine all the ketchup ingredients and blend until smooth and creamy. Add the water if needed for consistency. Makes 12 ounces

2. For the "fries": Cut the squash or jicama into French fry shapes. If using jicama, peel it first.

TOMATOES naturally contain an assortment of antioxidants, vitamins, and minerals than can actually prevent conditions including bone loss, diabetes, kidney stones, stroke, heart attack, cancer, and obesity.

YELLOW SUMMER SQUASH "FRIES" contain about 36 calories per cup. If you are trying to lose weight, yellow squash is a great choice to replace higher-calorie vegetables like potatoes. This little squash is also an amazing source of vitamin C and a very good source of vitamin A, magnesium, fiber, folate, copper, riboflavin, phosphorus, potassium, and manganese. Save the nutrients, eat your squash RAW!

CRUNCHY RAW JICAMA "FRIES" contain about 49 calories per cup. Eating jicama may improve the look of your skin, thanks to this vegetable's vitamin C content. The vitamin C you take in from eating jicama and other vitamin C-rich foods boosts collagen production. Not only does collagen improve the texture of your skin, but it also speeds wound healing, giving your skin a healthy appearance.

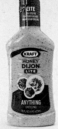

5

KRAFT HONEY DIJON SALAD DRESSING

Artificial food colors and dyes are all over our grocery store shelves—especially those products marketed to children. Parents don't think twice about feeding their kids fluorescent blue "juice," bright-orange cheese puffs, or rainbow-colored candies and cereals. The more color, the more danger.

Studies have been done on rats given doses of artificial food coloring versus a placebo and then placed in a maze. It was found that the rats were hyperactive and had difficulty staying on task and retaining attention. Most artificial brightly colored foods also have a lot of sugar, and people will blame the sugar on their child's hyperactivity. However, the coloring itself may have something to do with this as well. If your child already has trouble paying attention, such as with ADD or ADHD, consider whether coloring might be worsening their behavior.

Ingredients: Water, Soybean(s) Oil, Honey, Mustard Dijon (Vinegar, Mustard Seed, Salt, Water, Wine White, Spice(s), Vinegar, Sugar, Corn Syrup, contains less than 22% of Salt, Garlic Juice, Onion(s) Juice, Xanthan Gum, Citric Acid, Propylene Glycol Alginate, Caramel Color, Spice(s), Flavor(s) Natural, Phosphoric Acid, Vitamin E, **Yellow #5, Yellow #6**.

CREAMY HONEY MUSTARD DRESSING

I have always loved a Creamy Honey Mustard Dressing. Enjoy this dressing on any salad or serve as a dip with romaine Chips (page 15).

2 cups raw cashews

1¼ cups olive oil

¾ cup fresh lemon juice

3 small garlic cloves

2 teaspoons salt

¾ cup water

2 tablespoons apple cider vinegar

2 to 3 tablespoons raw honey, to taste

1 tablespoon Dijon mustard

1 teaspoon chopped chives, for garnish, optional

In a high-speed blender, combine all the ingredients and blend until smooth. Garnish with fresh chives, if using.

MAKES 36 OUNCES

INCREASE COPPER INTAKE

Cashews are one of the best sources for dietary copper. You need copper for proper brain function. Copper is involved in the production and secretion of dopamine and melanin. Without enough copper, you can develop chronic fatigue syndrome, depression, and other neurological disorders.

Failing to include sufficient copper in your diet can lead to low melanin production, which can cause prematurely gray hair. Cashews may be your color fix. Dietary copper is great for breaking down the fat in your food. Inadequate copper intake can raise your blood triglycerides and increase your risk of fatty liver and heart disease.

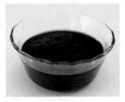

6

THAI KITCHEN PEANUT SATAY SAUCE

One in 25 school-age children has allergies to peanuts. This is why so many schools today have banned peanuts. For those with severe allergies, peanuts can cause the body to go into anaphylactic shock, a life-threatening condition where a person's blood pressure drops and airways narrow.

Ingredients: **Peanuts**, Coconut, Unrefined Cane Sugar, Soybean Oil, Lemon Grass, Garlic, Chili, Onion, Sesame, Salt, Galangal, Citric Acid, Lime, Xantham Gum.

NOT PEANUT SAUCE*

*No peanuts harmed in this recipe

Not Peanut Sauce was the very first dressing I ever created. I think I ate this dressing for a year until I felt confident enough to branch out and try something new. It's a good one. This sauce is thick and creamy, which makes it very satisfying and a good choice for those moving from a traditional heavy cooked diet into a lighter raw diet. Not Peanut Sauce is great with Spring Rolls (page 100).

Peanuts have a naturally occurring mold and that is why so many people are sensitive to them. I use a raw almond butter instead.

1 cup raw almond butter	3 tablespoons tamari
½ cup water	¼ cup olive oil
¼ cup fresh lemon juice	3 small garlic cloves
3 to 4 tablespoons peeled and chopped fresh ginger	½ serrano pepper, cut and seeded (check the heat of your pepper and adjust to taste)
¼ cup Grade B maple syrup	

In a blender, combine all the ingredients and blend. You can always add more water if you feel this dressing is too thick for you.

MAKES 23 OUNCES

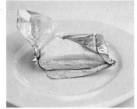

7

COMMERCIALLY PACKAGED CREAM CHEESE

The problem with the cream cheese coming from the dairy industry is that most of the time cows are treated inhumanely while being pumped full of antibiotics and growth hormones. Then after that, the milk is homogenized and pasteurized, making it a lifeless food source. We deserve better food than this.

BASIC WHITE SAUCE . . .
THE PERFECT CREAM CHEEZE

This sauce is so simple, yet so versatile—it is "the little black dress" of sauces. I make a thick version for a ricotta cheese or a cream cheese consistency. A slightly thinner version makes for a simple sour cream or dressing base. This sauce stands well alone, or you can add in favorite spices and flavors creating a unique dipping sauce or cream cheese tailored for you.

2 cups raw cashews	⅔ to 1 cup water
1 cup olive oil	2 teaspoons salt
¾ cup fresh lemon juice	3 small garlic cloves

In a high-speed blender, combine all the ingredients, using ⅔ cup water for a cream cheese consistency or 1 cup water for a sauce consistency. Store in the refrigerator, where it will thicken. Simply add more water if you need to thin it out for future recipes.

MAKES 30 OUNCES

HEART-PROTECTIVE MONOUNSATURATED FATS

Approximately 75% of the cashew's fat is unsaturated fatty acids, plus about 75% of this unsaturated fatty acid content is oleic acid, the same heart-healthy monounsaturated fat found in olive oil. Studies have shown that oleic acid promotes good cardiovascular health. Monounsaturated fat, when added to the low-fat diet of diabetic patients, actually helps lower triglyceride levels. So enjoy your cashews, especially if you have diabetes.

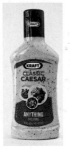

8

KRAFT CLASSIC CAESAR SALAD DRESSING

This bottled dressing gets a Big Fat F in my opinion. Not much here sounds like real food.

Ingredients: Water, Soybean(s) Oil, Vinegar, Cheese Parmesan and, Cheese Romano From Cows Milk (Milk Part Skim, Cheese Cultures, Salt, Enzyme(s)), Salt, contains less than 22% of Egg(s) Yolks, Garlic Juice, Food Starch Modified, Sugar, Xanthan Gum, Lactic Acid, Soy Protein Hydrolyzed, Corn Syrup Dried, with Sorbic Acid and, Calcium Disodium **EDTA** as Preservatives, Spice(s), Phosphoric Acid, Polysorbate 60, Fish Anchovies, Onion(s) Green Dried, Caramel Color, Parsley Dried, Color(s) Artificial, Garlic Dried, Soy Flour Defatted, Cottonseed Oil Partially Hydrogenated and/or Soybean(s) Oil Partially Hydrogenated, Soybean(s), Tamarind, Wheat, Yellow #5, Flavor(s) Natural.

THE CHAMPION CAESAR SALAD DRESSING

The Power of Words and Believing in Myself

My favorite salad of all time has always been Caesar Salad. I love that creamy Parmesan cheese taste with crispy romaine. Throughout my travels, I created amazing dishes for my families, but the perfect Caesar continued to elude me. I just couldn't create this seemingly simple dressing. I finally diagnosed the problem . . . it was my language of using the words "I can't." Then and there I announced, "I will create the best Caesar Salad ever!" I changed "I can't" to "I will!" and I did it!

The very next day in a class I was teaching, I heard the word "Caesar." My ears perked up and after class I headed over to my newfound friend, Elizabeth Champion. She offered to share her family's beloved secret Caesar dressing recipe with me. Since her boys plan on bottling this dressing and making millions, I will

WHAT IS EDTA?

EDTA (ethylenediaminetetraacetic acid) is one of the most powerful metal chelators known. It's a chemical that neutralizes bits of metal that are in the dressing from the factory's pipes and machines used in its production. It is added so the metal does not deteriorate the ingredients as they spend their long shelf-lives together.

We are adding chemicals to our foods in order to destroy chemicals in our foods!

not share this recipe with you, but with a little innovative thinking and some modifications, I was finally able to create a nondairy raw version that I am so proud to share with you and even happier to eat myself! Thank you, Elizabeth, for the inspiration.

Thanks to the power of words, you are about to enjoy the Champion Caesar dressing! I like to toss this dressing with romaine and top with tomato, fermented gingered carrots, and avocado slices.

2 organic eggs (choose eggs with no cracks, wash the outer shells with soap and water before cracking)

¼ cup apple cider vinegar

3 tablespoons fresh lemon juice

1 or 2 small garlic cloves, to taste

¾ teaspoon salt

1 cup olive oil

Fresh cracked black pepper

In a high-speed blender, combine the eggs, vinegar, lemon juice, garlic, and salt and blend everything at a medium speed (level 7 on a Vitamix) for about 30 seconds. Keep the blender going and slowly pour in the oil. The pouring should take you 60 seconds . . . that is slow pouring. Now turn the blending speed to high for about another 20 seconds until the dressing is thick and creamy. Sprinkle in pepper to taste and blend lightly.

MAKES 15 OUNCES

DRESS UP YOUR GREENS

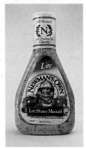

9

NEWMAN'S OWN® LITE HONEY MUSTARD DRESSING

Maltodextrin is a processed food additive that is not necessary in our foods. Even though food manufacturers and the FDA list it as being "natural," it is not found as an isolate in nature. Maltodextrin is created in a lab, not a kitchen.

Ingredients: Water, Creole Mustard (Ground Mustard Seed, Distilled Vinegar, Salt), Cider Vinegar, Sugar, Vegetable Oil (Soybean Oil and/or Canola Oil), **Maltodextrin,** Honey, Contains 2% or less of: Salt, Buttermilk Solids (Milk), Spice, Xanthan Gum, Lemon Juice Concentrate, Onion, Garlic.

HONEY'S DIJON VINAIGRETTE

This has become a favorite dressing of mine, especially because it is not made *by* me, but *for* me. This is my husband's creation, and when I come home from weeks of travel, he will often have this one prepared just for me.

1 cup olive oil	3 tablespoons raw honey
½ cup apple cider vinegar	¼ teaspoon salt
2 tablespoons Dijon mustard	Freshly ground black pepper, to taste

In a blender, combine all the ingredients and blend. Wow!!! That was easy. Serve to *your* honey.

MAKES 15 OUNCES

APPLE CIDER VINEGAR

When it comes to vinegars, I always choose apple cider vinegar. It is the only vinegar that does not turn acidic in the body. Our bodies are supposed to be slightly more alkaline, but a poor diet and lifestyle habits create in us an acidic state. This is what sets us up for weight gain, pain in the body, and illness. Apple cider vinegar, along with plenty of raw fruits and vegetables, helps us restore our body's proper pH level.

Apple cider vinegar also aids in weight loss by stabilizing the blood sugar and controlling the appetite. Try taking 1 to 2 teaspoons before each meal. Don't fool yourself though; if your diet is complete rubbish, apple cider vinegar is not going to miraculously trim you down. It should be accompanied by a healthy, balanced diet, rich in fresh fruits and vegetables . . . preferably *raw*.

To get the most health benefits from your apple cider vinegar, choose a raw, unfiltered, unpasteurized, organic brand.

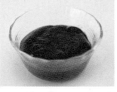

10

KIKKOMAN THAI YELLOW CURRY SAUCE

Raw Makeover 911 to the rescue!

Ingredients: Water, Coconut Milk Powder [Coconut Milk (Tree Nut), Maltodextrin, Sodium Caseinate (Milk)], Sugar, Yellow Thai Curry Paste (Red Chili, Garlic, Soybean Oil, Onion, Salt, Spices, Spice Extractives), Garlic, Green Thai Curry Paste [Green Chili, Onion, Salt, Garlic, Spices, Lemongrass, Galangal, Canola Oil, Dried Shrimp (Crustacean Shellfish), Spice Extractives], Contains 2% or less of the following: Soybean Oil, Fish Sauce (Anchovy Extract, Salt, Water), Modified Corn Starch, Salt, Onion, Dehydrated Onion, Citric Acid, Yeast Extract, Turmeric, Vinegar, Xanthan Gum, Alcohol (to preserve freshness).

AYURVEDA

Eating healthy can be delicious and gratifying, and that is the beauty of curry power. Ayurvedic medicine recognizes six flavors found in foods: sweet, sour, salty, bitter, astringent, and pungent. Because this curry sauce covers all six of these flavors, this dressing will completely satisfy, and you will eat much less.

Indian curry powder contains a number of ingredients, and every curry powder recipe is unique. A few of my favorite ingredients are cumin and coriander, which are helpful for digestion and conditions like irritable bowel syndrome, gas, and bloating. Also found in curry powder, turmeric is an antioxidant and anti-inflammatory.

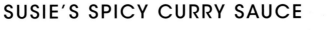

SUSIE'S SPICY CURRY SAUCE

Growing up in the South, I never ate curry. This new flavor that I found in a Chicago family's home intrigued me. I began to play with curry and created this delightful sauce, perfect for dressing a cole slaw or used as a dipping sauce!

¼ cup olive oil

¼ cup tamari

2 tablespoons apple cider vinegar

2 tablespoons fresh lemon juice

2 tablespoons raw honey

2 small garlic cloves

1-inch piece of fresh ginger

1 tablespoon curry powder

1 teaspoon chili powder

¼ to ½ serrano or jalapeño pepper, cut and seeded (test the heat of your pepper and adjust to taste)

In a blender, combine all the ingredients and blend until smooth.

MAKES 9 OUNCES

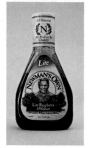

NEWMAN'S OWN® LITE RASPBERRY & WALNUT DRESSING

Refined sugar comes from sugar beet or sugar cane that has been stripped of all nutritional value. This sugar is void of all minerals, vitamins, and proteins. Your body gets a carbohydrate boost but absolutely no other benefit from eating refined sugar except for a sugar high and a spike in your insulin. Your body actually has to utilize the good stuff, like potassium, calcium, sodium, and magnesium, in order to metabolize these empty calories.

Ingredients: Water, **Sugar**, Vegetable Oil (Soybean Oil and/or Canola Oil), Red Wine Vinegar, Corn Syrup Solids, Contains 2% or less of: Raspberry, Walnuts, Salt, Natural Flavor, Orange Juice Concentrate, Onion, Xanthan Gum, Garlic, Spices, Natural Elderberry Extract and Annatto (for color).

HONEY GIRL'S STRAWBERRY VINAIGRETTE

Honey Girl, we did it! We shopped, prepared, styled, and photographed! Thank you so much for coming into my life, Karen. Thank you for the opportunity to feed you, your family, friends, and community. We started out as strangers and quickly became forever friends! A huge thank you to Shawn, Ocean (for giving me his bedroom), and North for being such a dreamy family. I love you all so very much. This dressing is *yours*, my dears.

1 cup strawberries	1 teaspoon salt
½ cup apple cider vinegar	1 garlic clove
½ cup olive oil	2 tablespoons finely chopped scallions
½ cup raw honey	

In a high-speed blender, combine all the ingredients and blend until creamy.

MAKES 20 OUNCES

RAW HONEY

Raw honey is an alkaline-forming food that contains important nutrients, live enzymes, powerful antioxidants, and vitamins. Raw honey is great for strengthening the immune system, relieving allergies, and improving digestive health.

When shopping for raw honey, carefully read the labels. Look for the word RAW. Beware of the typical little grocery store plastic bear filled with processed honey. This is no better than refined sugar.

Note: It is recommended that children under one year of age not be given honey.

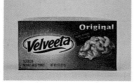

12

VELVEETA ROTEL CHEESE DIP

Many of us, at some point, have dipped into the popular Velveeta Rotel Cheese dip. Is this dip really cheese? Velveeta is classified as a "pasteurized prepared cheese product." Velveeta cannot legally call itself cheese. So what is it?

Ingredients: Milk, Water, Milkfat, Whey, Whey Protein Concentrate, Sodium Phosphate, Milk Protein Concentrate, Alginate, Sodium Citrate, Apocarotenal, Annatto, Enzymes, Benzoate, Cheese Culture.

NOT-CHO-CHEEZE SAUCE

The secret to re-creating families' favorite comfort foods is by capturing the essence with color, texture, and flavor. If you can pull these three things off, you can tell someone they are eating nacho cheese when actually they are eating some blended nuts and vegetables. My version combines some very distinct flavors that surprisingly taste like nacho cheese when blended! You will use this recipe for making Spicy Nori Nachos (page 67), Cheatos (page 61), and Cheezy Kale Chips (page 62). Top The Perfect Picnic Burger (page 90) and Firehouse Tostadas (page 86) with this delicious sauce, too. Or slice zucchini into round chips for quick and easy dipping!

1 orange, peeled
1 large red bell pepper, chopped
3 small garlic cloves
½ serrano or jalapeño pepper, cut and seeded (test

the heat of your pepper and adjust to taste)
2½ tablespoons fresh lemon juice
2 tablespoons tamari
2 cups raw cashews

In a high-speed blender, layer the orange segments and bell pepper at the bottom (this will make blending your cashews much easier). Then add the remaining ingredients and blend until smooth.

MAKES 24 OUNCES

EAT RED!

The color red has long been associated with passion, strength, and health. Fruits and vegetables in the red family (red bell peppers and oranges included) are known to prevent cardiovascular diseases, reduce risk of cancer, strengthen our immune systems, and help people with anemia, who are weak or vulnerable to viruses. Red fruits and vegetables contain lycopene and anthocyanin, which helps our bodies fight of disease. The phytochemicals in these red fruits and vegetables have antiaging benefits as well.

13

RAGÚ OLD WORLD STYLE TRADITIONAL PASTA SAUCE

You may be tempted to opt for this "light" sauce because it comes in at 35 calories for ¼ cup. Though it may be low in calories, it also comes in low on the healing benefits because it has been cooked. Raw pasta sauce, on the other hand, is packed full of fresh ingredients and live enzymes. These live enzymes are known healers. The fresh ingredients in raw sauces are always going to be better for you than a product that can sit on a shelf for a year . . . or more.

Ingredients: Tomato Puree (Water, Tomato Paste), Soybean Oil, Salt, Sugar, Dehydrated Onions, Extra Virgin Olive Oil, Spices, Romano Cheese (Part-Skim Milk, Cheese Cultures, Salt, Enzymes), Natural Flavor.

LYCOPENE

Study after study has concluded that eating more tomatoes may lower risks of certain types of cancers, especially prostate, lung, and stomach cancers. It is an important substance called lycopene (which gives the tomato its red color) that helps prevent these cancers.

Many conclude that processed tomatoes contain more lycopene than raw tomatoes. They say this is because processing, or cooking, breaks down the cell walls, helping to release the lycopene. The good news is, blending your raw tomatoes also releases lycopene! Eating raw tomatoes with some fat, such as a cold-pressed olive oil, helps lycopene to be better absorbed by the body.

TYRANNOSAURUS RED SAUCE

Everyone loves this raw marinara sauce. Every family I have visited has had a hand in creating this sauce. I especially thank all my Italian families for their input and for giving me the thumbs up. The final missing ingredient came from a family on Martha's Vineyard. I was complaining to my friend Rex that my sauce was not coming out *red* enough. He reminded me that I had used a *red* bell pepper to add color to my raw Not-Cho-Cheeze (page 32), so why not add a red bell pepper to my marinara sauce? Brilliant! I added the pepper and my sauce was complete. This sauce took me a year to finalize and I am so proud to share it with you all. Thank you, Rex!

Serve the sauce over raw zucchini noodles one night and save the leftovers for making Raw Pizzas (page 81) or Lasagna (page 83).

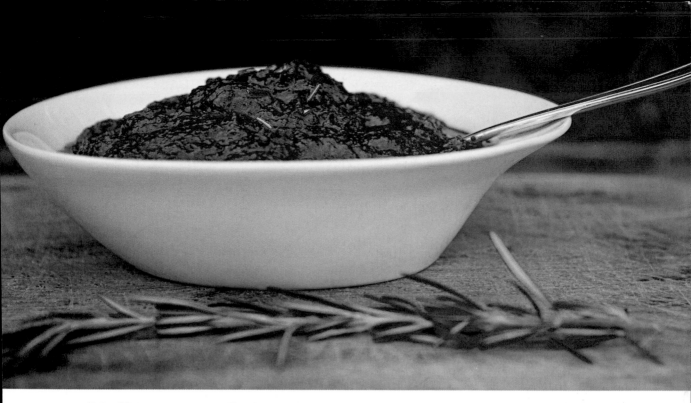

Note: This sauce is totally dependent on the quality of your fresh tomatoes. Pick organic tomatoes in season. You will be amazed! If your tomatoes are out of season, or a bit lacking, try adding an additional date or two. Also helpful would be some garlic salt to taste.

4 cups chopped tomatoes	2 tablespoons Italian herb seasoning
1 red bell pepper	1 teaspoon salt
3 small garlic cloves	½ cup oil-packed sun-dried tomatoes, drained
½ cup olive oil	⅓ cup chopped red onion
2 tablespoons fresh lemon juice	½ serrano or jalapeño pepper, cut and seeded (test
1 to 2 pitted dates	the heat of your pepper and adjust to taste)

1. There are two family versions for preparing your marinara.

2. **Family Favorite #1:** Some families like a creamy consistency. For this version, simply blend all the ingredients in a blender.

3. **Family Favorite #2:** If your family likes a chunkier version, put the ingredients into your food processor and pulse.

MAKES 56 OUNCES

DRESS UP YOUR GREENS

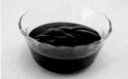

14

KIKKOMAN TERIYAKI MARINADE AND SAUCE

Kikkoman teriyaki sauce is a blend of high fructose corn syrup, some soy sauce, a dash of succinic acid, and a smidge of sodium benzoate.

What is succinic acid? Succinic acid is a four carbon dicarboxylic acid used in clothing fibers, surfactants, detergents, fragrances, and flavors. It serves as a starting material for a number of chemicals used in the pharmaceutical industry. Succinic acid is used as an acidity regulator, preservative, and flavor enhancer in our foods.

The nice thing about eating in-season vegetables and fruits: Your acidity levels are naturally regulated and the flavors are the richest in their freshly picked state. No succinic acid necessary.

Ingredients: Naturally Brewed Soy Sauce (Water, Wheat, Soybeans, Salt), Wine, **High Fructose Corn Syrup**, Water, Vinegar, Salt, Spices, Onion Powder, **Succinic Acid**, Garlic Powder, **Sodium Benzoate**: less than $\frac{1}{10}$ of 1% as a preservative.

~⤳

SUPER SIMPLE MARINADE

This super simple marinade is as perfect as it sounds. Trust me, you can't go wrong! You can marinate and dehydrate all kinds of vegetables for a nice vegetable "sauté." I use these marinated and dehydrated vegetables for Fajitas (page 94) and the China Bowl (page 96). Best part is you keep all the enzymes and nutrients ALIVE!

I eyeball the measurements, using the main 3 ingredients in these proportions: 2 parts olive oil, 1 part tamari, 1 part apple cider vinegar or lemon juice. Now, if you really must measure, and you want to get a little fancy with the Super Simple Marinade, here is a great place to begin.

½ cup olive oil	1 tablespoon raw honey
¼ cup tamari	1-inch piece of fresh ginger
¼ cup apple cider vinegar	2 small garlic cloves
1½ tablespoons fresh lemon juice	*Optional*: Dried red chile or red pepper flakes

In a high-speed blender, combine all the ingredients and blend until smooth—yummiest marinade or dressing at the press of a button.

MAKES 10 OUNCES

EAT RAW, NOT COOKED

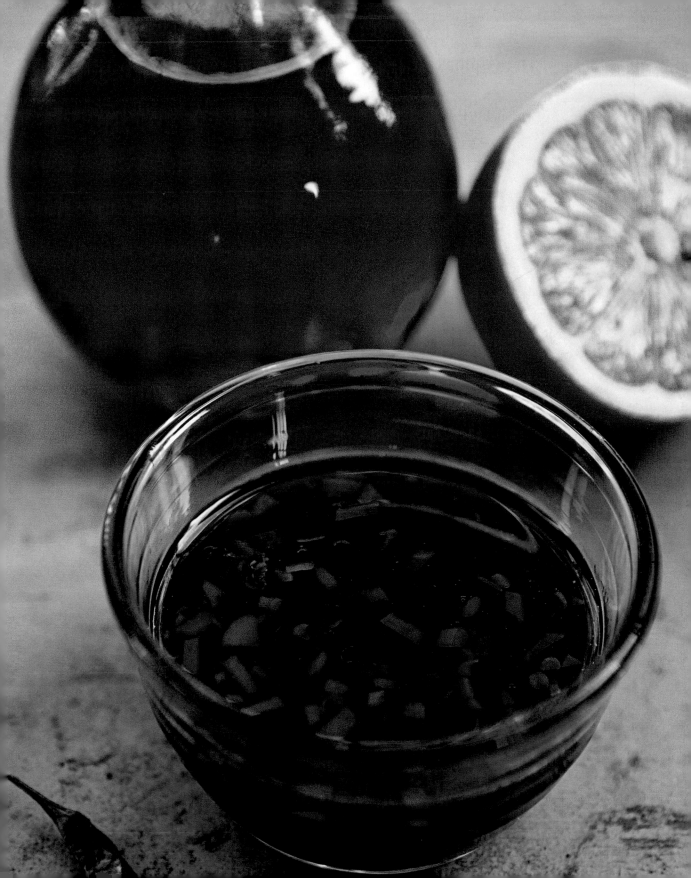

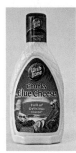

15

WISH-BONE® CHUNKY BLUE CHEESE SALAD DRESSING

Hydrogenated oils like "partially hydrogenated soybean oil" will fatten you up and eventually kill you. Hydrogenation is a process of heating oil and passing bubbles through it. The fatty acids in the oil acquire some of the hydrogen, which thickens it like butter. This thick oil gives processed foods a rich texture and flavor, while being cheap to produce. Before Americans started becoming epidemically fat, food producers had used coconut oil to get this rich buttery texture and flavor. Times changed, wallets tightened, and hydrogenated oils came on the scene.

Ingredients: Soybean Oil, Water, Whey, **Partially Hydrogenated Soybean and Cottonseed Oils**, Blue Cheese (Pasteurized Milk, Cheese, Cultures, Salt, Enzymes, Calcium Chloride), Maltodextrin, contains less than 2% of Egg Yolk, Natural Flavors, White Wine Vinegar, Distilled Vinegar, High Fructose Corn Syrup, Yeast Extract, Onion, Spice, Modified Food Starch, Salt, Whey Protein Concentrate, Lactic Acid, Phosphoric Acid, Xanthan Gum, Polysorbate 60, Disodium Inosinate, Disodium Guanylate, Artificial Flavor, Sorbic Acid, Sodium Benzoate and Calcium Disodium EDTA (to preserve freshness).

NOT BLUE CHEESE DRESSING

Definitely not Blue Cheese Dressing, this is an edgy dressing with a punch, that will soon replace your bottled blue cheese dressing. This dressing was inspired by my dear friend Lynne McLaine. Lynne has a family history of heart disease and has been on blood pressure medication since she was a teenager. She knew if she didn't gain control of her health proactively she might eventually fall victim to some of the same things many of her family members had early in life. Lynne loves a good challenge and so she took on a 30-Day Raw Food Challenge!

Now completely off medications, Lynne says, "Those 30 days dramatically changed my life in ways that even today I find hard to articulate, but

> ### MAD FOR MACADAMIAS
>
> Macadamia nuts are a great source of magnesium, potassium, calcium, iron, and fiber. They contain selenium, which is a natural antioxidant that may help reduce certain types of cancers. Macadamia nuts are rich tasting along with being cholesterol free.

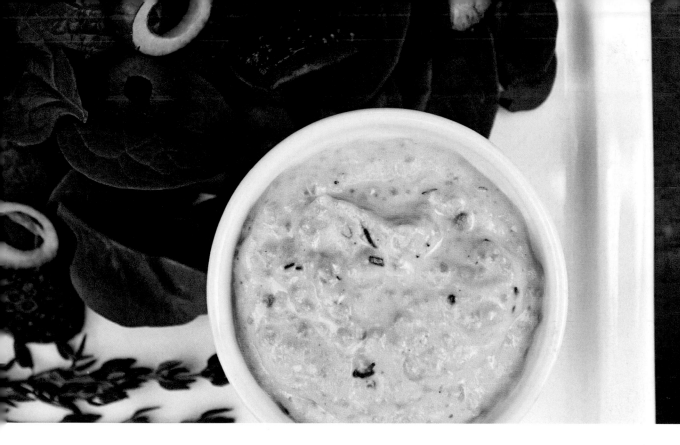

that doesn't stop me from trying!" Today Lynne has a zest for life that radiates as she shares her new passion for raw foods!

1 cup macadamia nuts

¼ cup scallions

¼ cup red onion

1½ cups Basic White Sauce (page 22), made to a thick dressing consistency using about 1 cup water

⅓ cup apple cider vinegar (the "edge"—feel free to add more or less "edge" according to your taste)

1 teaspoon sea salt

½ teaspoon freshly ground black pepper

½ tablespoon finely chopped fresh thyme leaves

½ tablespoon finely chopped fresh rosemary

1. In a food processor, combine the macadamia nuts, scallions, and onion and process until coarsely chopped. Add the Basic White Sauce and vinegar and pulse until lightly blended.

2. Transfer to a bowl and stir in the salt, pepper, thyme, and rosemary.

MAKES 16 OUNCES

DRESS UP YOUR GREENS

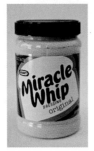

16

WHAT'S IN YOUR COLESLAW?

Many popular coleslaw recipes call for a dressing of Miracle Whip, vinegar, and sugar. What is Miracle Whip? A white dressing similar to mayonnaise, but less expensive. Miracle Whip has been a huge hit and very popular with many Americans. It's time to ask ourselves: Is it real food?

Soybean oil makes up the majority of Miracle Whip's ingredients. Back in the '90s, food manufacturers began being forced by the FDA to label the trans fat content on their products. To avoid any drop in sales, manufacturers started using soybean oil because it is a vegetable oil with no trans fat. What an easy fix, right? Not so easy. When you heat and process these vegetable oils, the molecular structure is changed, they become rancid, and damaging to our bodies at a cellular level. You are no better off than eating trans fats.

Miracle Whip Ingredients: Water, **Soybean Oil,** Glucose-Fructose, Vinegar, Sugar, Modified Cornstarch, Salt, Whole Egg, Egg Yolk, Corn Dextrin, Mustard, Color, Microcrystalline Cellulose, Potassium Sorbate, Spices, Xanthan Gum, Calcium Disodium EDTA, Dried Garlic, Modified Coconut Oil or Modified Palm Kernel Oil.

WICKED COLE SLAW DRESSING

What's up with all the coleslaw in New England? It's everywhere! I believe it's the New England National Salad. I have never liked coleslaw, but ever since re-creating it for my families, I now *looooove* coleslaw. As they say up north, it's "wicked"! This will make 4 cups, but it is so delicious that you won't want any less. It will store well and you can use it on any type of salad or as a dip for "Chips" & Dip (page 15). You may need to thin out this dressing with water as it thickens in the refrigerator.

2 cups raw cashews

1¼ cups olive oil

¾ cup fresh lemon juice

3 small garlic cloves

2 teaspoons salt

¾ cup water

6 tablespoons apple cider vinegar, or to taste

4 tablespoons raw agave nectar or raw honey, or to taste

In a high-speed blender, combine all the ingredients and blend until smooth.

MAKES 4 CUPS

EAT RAW, NOT COOKED

STACY'S WICKED SLAW

1 small cabbage (about 2 pounds)

Wicked Cole Slaw Dressing (page 40)

4 scallions, thinly sliced

6 radishes, thinly sliced

¼ cup flat-leaf parsley

2 avocados

Fresh cracked black pepper

Remove the outer leaves from the cabbage and cut out the core. Thinly slice the cabbage and coat with the dressing. Garnish with the scallions, radishes, parsley, avocados, and pepper to taste.

SERVES 4 TO 6

GROW YOUNGER ON CABBAGE

One cup of raw cabbage has only 22 calories, 0g fat, and 2g fiber. Cabbage is rich in Vitamin C (25.6mg of vitamin C for 1 cup of shredded cabbage). Vitamin C is one of the best antioxidants, reducing free radicals in the body. These free radicals are responsible for aging us quickly and must be stopped!

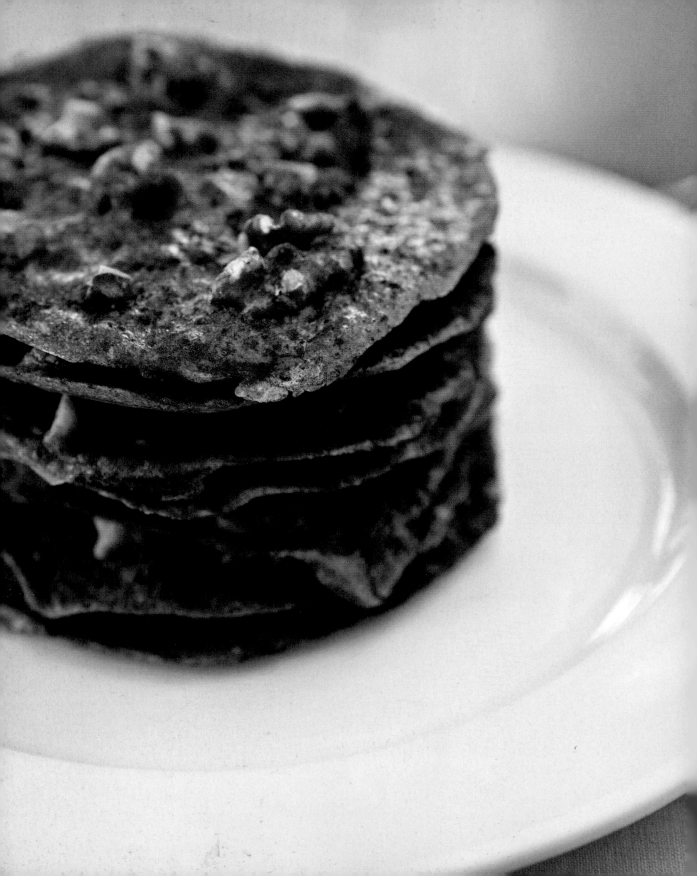

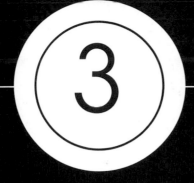

The Bakery

BREADS, CRACKERS, AND SNACKS

The Flagel

Cranberry-Orange Flagels

Chocolate-Frosted "Donut"

Banana Pancakes

Baby Grahams

Seeds of Change

Tostadas or Corn Chips

Cheatos

Cheezy Kale Chips

Sweet Tangy Kale Chips

Spicy Nori Nachos

Onion Rings

Not Fried, Not Clams

In this section, we are not actually baking, but it sure will taste like we are. I am able to reinvent a lot of family favorites using a dehydrator. Pretty soon, you will be making breads, chips, and tasty snacks, like my famous Cheatos (page 61)!

A dehydrator heats foods at a very low temperature. I dehydrate at 115°F. Heat much higher than that and you will start to destroy the nutrients and the enzymes in your foods. So I keep it low. This simply takes out the moisture in foods and makes them crispy—a texture we all crave.

Plan ahead when preparing for meals. Most things take 12 to 24 hours of drying time in the dehydrator. Drying times will always vary depending on your climate or how full your dehydrator is. The drying times I give you here are general estimates. Every kitchen, dehydrator, and weather condition seems to have a different drying time. Times will also vary because each chef will slice, layer, or pour batters at a different thickness. There is no harm in simply checking in on your creations from time to time. Just know one thing is for sure: Nothing ever burns in the dehydrator.

Dehydrated foods store well. I will sometimes throw things back into the dehydrator to crisp them up again after they have been stored, especially in a humid climate. This trick works wonders. I have snacked on cookies a month old! This is okay since there are no eggs, butter, or dairy used in these recipes to go bad.

▪ Flours ▪

You will be using various nuts, seeds, and grains to make flours in this section. This is really great for those who want to eliminate gluten from their diets. This also means you get a truly raw recipe full of rich live enzymes.

A nut "flour" is made from nuts that have been put in the freezer overnight and then ground in a food processor. Freezing the nuts first prevents them from turning into nut butter when you process them. Your "flour" will be similar in texture to coarse cornmeal. Grains do not have to be put in the freezer. Tiny seeds, like flaxseeds or sesame seeds, are best ground in a spice grinder or coffee grinder.

I love my Vitamix dry-grains attachment. This 32-ounce container is perfect for processing raw nuts, seeds, and grains into fresh "flours." Unlike with the food processor, you don't need to freeze the nuts beforehand.

THE BAGEL

What favorite food raises the blood sugar more than table sugar and candy bars? It's the good ole bagel, along with sandwich bread, pasta, baguettes, croissants, muffins, pizza crusts, crackers, donuts, pancakes, waffles, and cookies, rice and potatoes included. It doesn't matter if the bread is whole-grain, multigrain, stone-ground, or gluten-free. These starches give us a blood sugar high, leading to a blood sugar low, in turn causing us to crave even more bread and sugar before the first bite has even left our stomachs. This food is highly addictive, and we will cling to it like an addict until we are ready to let it go.

Instead, eat the richest foods on the planet. Fresh green leaves, salmon, and raw nuts will not raise your blood sugar. Eat these foods, along with all the many other colorful vegetables, fruits, seeds, and healthy oils there are to choose from when you are hungry.

The calories in a typical whole grain bagel will run you 400 calories. If you add just 1 ounce of cream cheese to that, you get another 100 calories, coming to a whopping 500 calories!

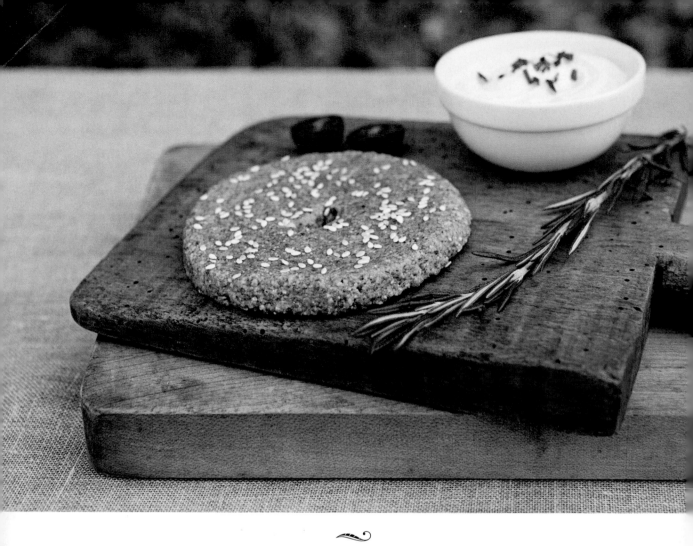

THE FLAGEL

What's a "flagel"? A flat bagel. These are so buttery tasting that unlike your typical bagel, you really won't miss the cream cheese or butter. Flagels are made out of farro, which can be found at many health food stores or ordered online as well. This recipe is not difficult. In fact it is extremely easy. If you remember how to play with Play-Doh, you will be a great flagel maker!

The flagel will run you 325 calories. Without the dramatic increase in blood sugar you get from a typical bagel, the flagel will keep you feeling satisfied longer.

3 cups farro, ground into flour

2 cups raw cashews, ground into flour

2 to 2½ cups raw almonds, ground into flour

2 teaspoons sea salt

1 can (13.5 ounces) organic coconut milk

2 tablespoons raw honey

1 tablespoon unrefined coconut oil

1. In a large bowl, mix together the farro flour, cashew flour, almond flour, and salt.

2. In a second bowl, combine the coconut milk, honey, and coconut oil.

3. Add the wet ingredients to the dry and combine the two mixtures by hand. The mixture should be a thick, moldable dough, like Play-Doh. Nothing too wet. (Note: If your dough is too wet, add a bit more nut flour of your choice or simply let your dough sit for about 15 minutes. The longer your dough sits the harder it will become, as the flours will absorb the moisture. On the other hand, if you have to leave your dough and it gets too dry, simply add some water when you return.)

4. Now channel your kindergarten Play-Doh shaping days. Take ¼ to ⅓ cup of dough (you get to choose your flagel size) and roll it into a ball. Form your ball into a log and shape the dough around into a bagel shape. Flatten your bagel into a flagel no thicker than ¼ inch thick.

5. Dehydrate for 24 hours at 115°F on unlined dehydrator trays (do not use nonstick sheets). This allows more air circulation and a quicker drying.

MAKES 15 TO 19 FLAGELS

FARRO WAY

Farro is a hearty, nutty grain long loved by the Italians. It won't spike blood sugar and is low in gluten, making it easy to digest, even on a gluten-free diet. Farro's complex carbohydrates break down slowly, keeping you energized, and its fiber content is a plus for filling us up, preventing colon cancer, and keeping us regular.

CRANBERRY-ORANGE FLAGELS

Flagels are so much fun to play with. I have experimented with everything from cinnamon-raisin to "Everything" Flagels. Be adventurous and come up with your own flavor profiles. My absolute favorite combination is cranberry-orange.

3 cups farro, ground into flour

2 cups raw cashews, ground into flour

2 to 2½ cups raw almonds, ground into flour

Grated zest from 2 oranges

1 cup dried cranberries

2 teaspoons sea salt

1½ cups canned organic coconut milk

¼ cup fresh orange juice

2 tablespoons raw honey

1 tablespoon unrefined coconut oil

1. In a large bowl, mix together the farro flour, cashew flour, almond flour, orange zest, craberries, and salt.

2. In a second bowl, combine the coconut milk, orange juice, honey, and coconut oil.

3. Add the wet ingredients to the dry and combine the two mixtures by hand. The mixture should be a thick, moldable dough, like Play-Doh. Nothing too wet. (Note: If your dough is too wet, add a bit more nut flour of your choice or simply let your dough sit for about 15 minutes. The longer your dough sits the harder it will become, as the flours will absorb the moisture. On the other hand, if you have to leave your dough and it gets too dry, simply add some water when you return.)

4. Now channel your kindergarten Play-Doh shaping days. Take ¼ to ⅓ cup of dough (you get to choose your flagel size) and roll it into a ball. Form your ball into a log and shape the dough around into a bagel shape. Flatten your bagel into a flagel no thicker than ¼ inch thick.

5. Dehydrate for 24 hours at 115°F on unlined dehydrator trays (do not use nonstick sheets). This allows more air circulation and a quicker drying.

MAKES 15 TO 19 FLAGELS

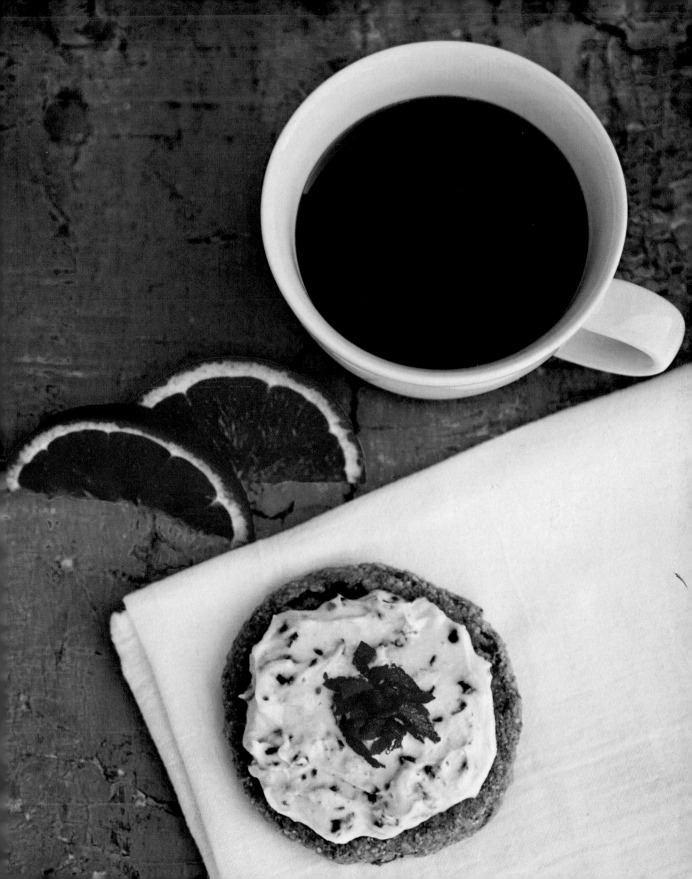

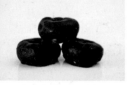

18

HOSTESS FROSTED DONETTES

A famous *SNL* skit stars a young John Belushi smoking a cigarette while crediting little chocolate donuts for his athletic success. Now that is humor! Even John knew back then how ridiculous a donut-filled breakfast was.

Ingredients: Sugar, Vegetable(s) Oil Partially Hydrogenated and/or, Animal Shortening contains one or more of the following (Soybean(s) Oil, Cottonseed Oil, Canola Oil, Palm Kernel Oil, Coconut Oil or, Palm Oil, Beef Fat), Wheat Flour Enriched (Flour, Barley Malt, Ferrous Sulfate [Iron], Vitamins [Niacin, Thiamine Mononitrate (Vitamin B1), Riboflavin (Vitamin B2), Folic Acid (Vitamin B9)]), Water, Cocoa, Cocoa Processed with Alkali, Soybean(s) Oil contains 2% or less of the Following: Milk Non-Fat, Soy Flour, Leavening (Sodium Acid Pyrophosphate, Baking Soda, Sodium Aluminum Phosphate), Egg(s) Yolks, Salt, Lecithin, Dextrose, Wheat Starch Modified, Mono and Diglycerides, Sorbitan Mono-stearate, Tapioca Dextrin, Corn Dextrins, Guar Gum, Karaya Gum, Corn Starch Modified, Cellulose Gum, Enzyme(s), Corn Starch, Citric Acid, Potassium Sorbate to retain freshness, **Propylene Glycol**, Sodium Propionate, Sorbic Acid, Turmeric (Color(s)), Wheat Starch, **Flavor(s) Natural & Artificial**, of Annatto Extracts.

In honor of John Belushi . . .

CHOCOLATE-FROSTED "DONUT"

What is better than a Flagel? A Flagel frosted in Chocolate Ganache!!!

Flagel (pages 46–47) + Chocolate Ganache (page 150) = Chocolate Frosted "Donut"

Note: Make your Ganache right before frosting your Flagels. The ganache will become very thick as it sits. If needed, simply thin out the Ganache with a little water for frosting.

GIRLS, EAT YOUR CHOCOLATE-FROSTED "DONUTS"!

Raw chocolate and farro are both super high in magnesium. Magnesium helps the body absorb calcium, leaving us with healthy bones and teeth. Magnesium also relieves symptoms of menopause and premenstrual syndrome, and minimizes the risk of premature labor. It is really important for stress relief.

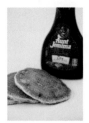

19

AUNT JEMIMA FROZEN BLUEBERRY PANCAKES AND SYRUP

Aunt Jemima has a rich history spanning over 120 years that gives off a feeling of warmth and nourishment for families. A staple item in many families' cabinets across the country, one has to wonder: What exactly is in this popular pancake and syrup combo?

Ingredients (pancakes): Enriched Wheat Flour (Flour, Niacin [Vitamin B3], Reduced Iron, Thiamin Mononitrate [Vitamin B1], Riboflavin [Vitamin B2], Folic Acid [Vitamin B9]), Nonfat Milk, Whey, Sugar, Blueberry Bits (Sugar, Dextrose, Soybean Oil, Soy Protein, Dried Blueberries, Natural Flavor, Cellulose Gum, Salt, Carrot Juice Extract [color], Blueberry Extract [color]), Whole Eggs, Water, Soybean Oil. Contains 2% or less of: Baking Powder (Baking Soda, Sodium Acid Pyrophosphate), Salt, Blueberry Puree Cornstarch, Vanilla Extract, Soy Flour. Contains: Wheat, Milk, Soy, Eggs.

Ingredients (Syrup): Corn Syrup, High Fructose Corn Syrup, Water, Cellulose Gum, Caramel Color, Salt, Sodium Benzoate and Sorbic Acid (Preservatives), Artificial and Natural Flavors, Sodium Hexametaphosphate.

DROP THE WHEAT, DROP THE WEIGHT

Wheat is very high in sugar. In fact, wheat increases our blood sugar levels just as much as a candy bar. Wheat, much like sugar, keeps us hungering for even more wheat. According to William Davis, MD, author of *Wheat Belly*, here are the changes that can occur when you cut out wheat:

- Flat abdomen
- Rapid weight loss
- High energy
- Few mood swings
- Better sleep
- Diminished appetite
- Reduced blood sugar

- Reduced blood pressure
- Reduced small LDL and total LDL
- Increased HDL cholesterol
- Reduced triglycerides
- Reduced C-reactive protein and other inflammatory measures

BANANA PANCAKES

These banana pancakes are sweet and yummy, made with bananas, walnuts, Grade B maple syrup, and cinnamon. After meeting a hyperactive three-year-old named Liam, who was accustomed to heavily processed sugars, juices, and wheat, I came up with these pancakes and he *loved* them. What an easy boy to feed! His mom was happy, and there were no more meltdowns on the floor of Target.

4 medium very-ripe bananas	2½ tablespoons Grade B maple syrup
½ cup chopped walnuts	Ground cinnamon

1. Set up a dehydrator and line the trays with nonstick sheets.

2. Blend the bananas in a blender. Pour ¼ cup blended bananas onto the sheets to make 3 ½-inch pancakes. Top with the walnuts. Drizzle on the maple syrup. Sprinkle with cinnamon to taste.

3. Dehydrate at 115°F for 12 hours. Peel the pancakes from the sheets and place them directly onto unlined dehydrator trays. Dehydrate 3 to 4 more hours if needed.

SERVINGS: 8 PANCAKES

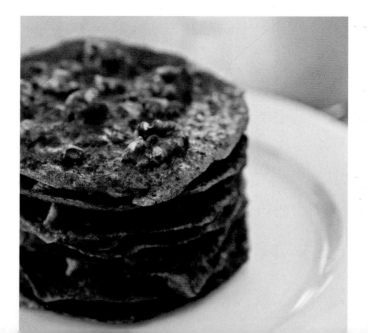

20

TEDDY GRAHAMS

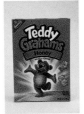

All across America, I see car seats and car floors scattered with the remnants of goldfish, pretzels, cereal, and graham cracker bears. Full of wheat, starches, and sugars, these foods are yet another highly processed food marketed to kids and busy parents. Be forewarned: This addictive, low-nutrient food will just leave your kids hungry for more sugary starches.

Ingredients: Graham Flour (Whole Grain Wheat Flour), Unbleached Enriched Flour (Wheat Flour, Niacin, Reduced Iron, Thiamine Mononitrate {Vitamin B1}, Riboflavin {Vitamin B2}, Folic Acid), Sugar, Soybean Oil, Dextrose, Maltodextrin, Calcium Carbonate (Source of Calcium), Baking Soda, Salt, Natural Flavor, Cinnamon, Soy Lecithin, Zinc Oxide (Source of Zinc), Reduced Iron.

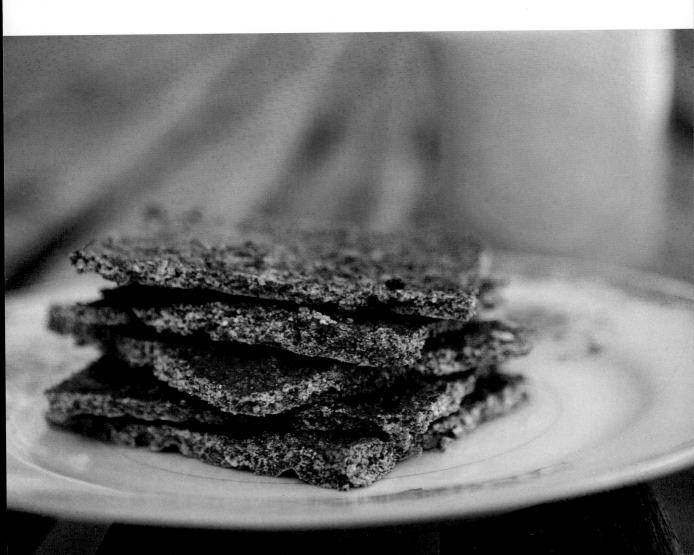

BABY GRAHAMS

One of the most common kids' snacks on playgrounds are graham crackers. But what if your child has so many allergies that the graham cracker just isn't an option? That was the case with the Shiu family. Not only did their youngest have a gluten allergy, she could not have dairy, nuts, or seeds. This really put me to the test. At first I thought, how in the world am I going to make a dairy-, gluten-, nut-, and seed-free graham cracker? Well, I did! Not only was my 2½ year old happy, *many* of my families LOVE this super simple graham cracker.

3 cups steel-cut oats, ground into flour
¾ cup raw coconut palm sugar, plus extra for dusting
¼ teaspoon sea salt

2 teaspoons pure vanilla extract
1 can (13.5 ounces) organic coconut milk
Ground cinnamon

1. Set up a dehydrator and line the trays with nonstick sheets.

2. In a high-speed blender, combine the oat flour, palm sugar, salt, vanilla, and coconut milk.

3. Spread the mixture onto the lined dehydrator trays ⅛ to ¼ inch thick. Sprinkle with palm sugar and cinnamon to taste. Dehydrate at 115°F for 8 to 10 hours or until dry to the touch. Flip and remove the liners. This would be a good time to cut into neat squares.

4. Continue to dry another 8 to 10 hours.

MAKES APPROXIMATELY 24 BABY GRAHAMS

OAT GROATS

I prefer using oat groats in place of the steel-cut oats when I can find a market that carries them. Oat groats are the least processed, but because they can be hard to find, I have called for steel-cut oats in this recipe.

STEEL-CUT OATS

Steel-cut oats are made by taking the groat and cutting it into tiny pieces using a steel blade. Because the steel-cut oat is not significantly processed, it has more nutrients than rolled oats, which are steamed, rolled, steamed again, and toasted.

Are steel-cut oats gluten free? Yes, steel-cut oats are gluten free if they have not been contaminated by machinery also handling other grains. To be completely safe, there are more and more companies offering gluten-free oats. To find this product, either check online or ask your grocer.

21

WHEAT THINS

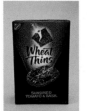

"Wheat" and "Thin"—whoever brought these two words together was a marketing wizard! I am told wheat is good, and I definitely wanna be thin. Jackpot!

"Wheat Fats" . . . there is a component to wheat called gliadin. Gliadin revs up our appetite and keeps us snacking throughout the day. Those of us who avoid wheat are not snacking every couple of hours. We eat fewer calories per day, and we avoid hydrogenated oils, high fructose corn syrups, preservatives, artificial flavorings, and colorings that typically come along with snack foods.

Ingredients: Whole Grain Wheat Flour, Unbleached Enriched Flour (Wheat Flour, Niacin, Reduced Iron, Thiamine Mononitrate {Vitamin B1}, Riboflavin {Vitamin B2}, Folic Acid), Soybean Oil, Sugar, Cornstarch, Malt Syrup (from Barley and Corn), Salt, Invert Sugar, Leavening (Calcium Phosphate and/or Baking Soda), Vegetable Color (Annatto Extract, Turmeric Oleoresin).

SEEDS OF CHANGE

This is a most amazing cracker! I also use it as a pizza crust. My friend Joan appropriately calls this cracker "Seeds of Change" in reference to the difference a raw food diet has made in her life. I sprinkle the top with King Arthur Everything Bread and Bagel Topping, a mixture of sesame seeds, poppy seeds, onion, garlic, and salt. Find it online at www.kingarthur.com.

1 cup sunflower seeds, ground into flour	1 tablespoon Italian herb seasoning
1 cup sesame seeds, ground into flour	1¼ teaspoons salt
1 cup flaxseeds, ground into flour (do not be tempted to substitute with preground flaxmeal)	½ cup water
½ cup chopped sweet onion	1 garlic clove, chopped
1 cup chopped tomato	Everything Bread and Bagel Topping

1. Set up a dehydrator and line the trays with nonstick sheets.

2. In a large bowl, toss together the ground seeds.

3. In a food processor or high-speed blender, blend the onion and tomato until liquefied. Blend in the Italian herbs, salt, water, and garlic. Pour this mixture into

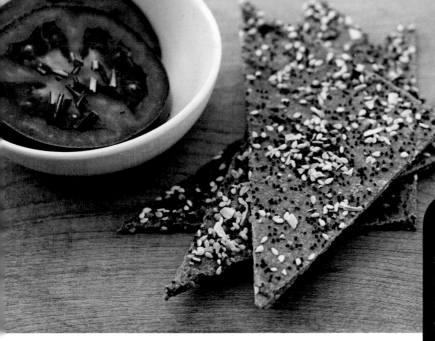

the ground seeds and stir. You may need to add more water; you want a sticky paste that holds together solidly and is the consistency of muffin batter.

4. Divide the batter into two portions. Spread onto the lined dehydrator trays ⅛ to ¼ inch thick. Sprinkle with the everything topping and dehydrate at 115°F for 8 hours. Flip the bread and remove the liners. This would be a good time to cut into neat sandwich-size squares or triangles.

5. Dehydrate another 8 hours or until desired dryness.

MAKES ABOUT 12 PIECES OF BREAD OR 48 TRIANGLE CRACKERS, OR 2 PIZZA CRUSTS CUT INTO 6 SLICES EACH

THE MIGHTY SEED

SUNFLOWER SEEDS: Perfect for those of us looking to lose weight, as these seeds promote healthy digestion and increase our fiber intake. They are full of crucial elements in preventing heart disease, cancer, and other forms of cellular damage, like vitamin E, selenium, and copper. Sunflower seeds are rich in folate, a very beneficial nutrient for women. So eat up, ladies!

SESAME SEEDS: Very high in calcium, iron, magnesium, zinc, fiber, phosphorus, and vitamin B1, studies have shown that sesame seeds can lower high blood pressure.

FLAXSEEDS: These seeds are high in most B vitamins, magnesium, manganese, and omega-3 fatty acids. Omega-3 fatty acids are key in fighting inflammation in our bodies. Inflammation plays a part in many chronic diseases, including diabetes, heart disease, arthritis, asthma, and even some cancers.

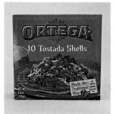

22

ORTEGA TOSTADA SHELLS

Hydrogenation of oils, with removal of essential fatty acids, is used in the food industry for the sole purpose of prolonging the shelf life of processed foods. They begin as natural healthy oils that quickly turn into poison once they have gone through processing. This is a slow poison that will sap your energy, store in fat, and lead to disease. Studies have linked the consumption of trans fats (hydrogenated and partially hydrogenated) found in many processed foods to the development of cancer, cardiovascular disease, and diabetes. Avoid these oils by eating fresh foods.

Ingredients: Corn Yellow, Soybean(s) Oil **Partially Hydrogenated**, Water, Salt, Corn Flour, Lime Hydrated.

TOSTADAS OR CORN CHIPS

This is a beautiful raw chip made out of corn, millet, and pumpkin seeds. I made this chip on a beautiful fall day when I was on a campaign to "save the pumpkin." I made pumpkin soup, pumpkin pie, and a raw corn chip using pumpkin seeds. The buttery yellow millet also adds the perfect color complement for these corn chips. The recipe makes either tostadas or chips (which are great dipped in Stacy's Guacamole, page 88). Ole!

2 bags (16 ounces each) frozen organic sweet corn, thawed

1½ cups pumpkin seeds

1½ to 2 cups millet, ground into flour

1 cup chopped sweet onion (1 medium onion)

¼ cup olive oil

2 tablespoons raw honey

2 teaspoons salt

1. In a food processor, combine the corn, pumpkin seeds, millet flour, onion, oil, honey, and salt and process until you get a thick batterlike mixture. If you have a smaller processor, you may need to either halve the recipe or do this in batches.

2. Set up a dehydrator and line the trays with nonstick sheets.

3. To make the tostadas, measure ¼ cup of the mixture for each and form a round onto the lined dehydrator trays, a little less than ¼ inch thick. Dehydrate at 115°F for 6 to 8 hours. Flip the tostadas and remove the liners. Continue to dehydrate for another 8 to 10 hours or until desired dryness.

4. To make the chips, follow the dehydrating instructions for the tostadas and when you flip and remove the liners, quarter the tostadas and continue with the dehydration.

MAKES 22 TOSTADA SHELLS OR 88 CORN CHIPS

THE HAPPY SEEDS

PUMPKIN SEEDS: These seeds are high in tryptophan, which is beneficial for reducing stress, improving sleep, and putting us in a happier mood. Deficiencies in tryptophan on the other hand are linked to trouble sleeping and depression.

MILLET: Tiny yellow seeds with a grainlike consistency, millet is gluten free and packed with essential vitamins and minerals. It is alkaline and digests easily. Millet keeps your colon hydrated and keeps you regular. Millet provides serotonin, which provides relief from stress. It does not feed yeast (candida). And it acts as a probiotic, stimulating microflora, feeding our inner ecosystems to keep us healthy and strong.

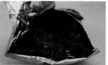

23

CHEETOS®

One Cheeto Addict's Plea . . .

Every day I swear I need Cheetos, either the super spicy kind or the puffed kind. How do I get away from this craving? Usually it's easy for me to avoid junk food, but OMG Cheetos are like crack for me. Eating healthy is way more appetizing, but I just can't get Cheetos out of my life! Why are some cravings so hard to ignore?

Signed,

Cheeto Addict

Dear Cheeto Addict,

Food manufacturers have been steadily increasing the amounts of "excitotoxins" in our foods, triggering an insulin, adrenalin, fat-storage, food-craving response. That response is what is causing you to head to your local 7-Eleven at midnight in your pajama pants, oversize hoodie, and baseball cap.

Beware of these ingredients and avoid at all cost: monopotassium glutamate, hydrolyzed plant protein, autolyzed plant protein, glutamic acid, sodium caseinate, autolyzed yeast, textured protein, gelatin, calcium caseinate. Even some so-called natural or healthy foods contain monosodium glutamate labeled as "yeast extract."

Love,

Stacy

Thinking back to my young junk food–loving days, the first thing that comes to mind are Cheetos. It was 1981 and I was thirteen when my Cheeto addiction began. If you don't know what a Cheeto is, it is this little cheesy curly crunchy thing that turns everything orange, and for a kid, that just made them even more desirable.

In 2010 I reinvented my favorite childhood snack for a picky nine year old I was trying to impress. I call them "Cheatos." I got a thumbs-up from the nine year old and I get to indulge in an old childhood favorite while "cheating" the negative effects of eating a highly processed junk food.

Ingredients: Enriched Corn Meal (Corn Meal, Ferrous Sulfate, Niacin, Thiamin Monoitrate, Riboflavin, and Frolic Acid), Vegetable Oil (Contains one or more of the following: corn, soybean, or sunflower oil), Whey, Salt, Cheddar Cheese, (Cultured Milk, Salt, Enzymes). Partially Hydrogenated Soybean Oil, Maltodextrin, Disodium Phosphate, Sour Cream (Cultured Cream, Nonfat Milk), Artificial Flavor, Monosodium Glutmate, Lactic Acid, Artificial Colors (Including Yellow 6), and Citric Acid.

CHEATOS

The Not-Cho-Cheeze Sauce is a batter for coating 2 medium heads of cauliflower pieces. You can always use one head of cauliflower and save the rest of your sauce for some Cheezy Kale Chips (page 62). Cauliflower is a beneficial food to eat when you are sick because it is rich in glutathione, a powerful antioxidant that helps to ward off infection. Move over, chicken noodle soup. . . .

2 medium heads cauliflower

Not-Cho-Cheeze Sauce (page 32), made without the chile pepper

1. Clean and cut the cauliflower into pieces the size of a Lego or a Barbie doll shoe. Coat the pieces in the Not-Cho-Cheeze Sauce.

2. Set up a dehydrator and line the trays with nonstick sheets.

3. Place a layer of coated cauliflower pieces onto the lined dehydrator tray. Fill as many trays as you desire. Dehydrate at 115°F for 6 hours. When dry to the touch, remove the liners and place the Cheatos onto the unlined trays. Dehydrate for another 6 to 8 hours. When they are crunchy, they are done. If they lose their crunch while being stored, simply put them back in the dehydrator for a few hours.

SERVES 6

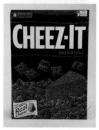

24

CHEEZ-ITS

Wheat plus chemically altered oils ensure you will be able to finish a box of Cheez-Its in a day. The low nutritional value will keep your body hungry, and the fatty taste in your mouth will have you craving more, more, more. It is almost a guarantee: You will need to chase these little orange wheat bombs down with a few diet sodas. The caffeine will hide the fog in your head, and the chemical sweetener will give your mouth a much-needed break from all the salt intake.

Ingredients: Enriched Flour (**Wheat Flour**, Niacin, Reduced Iron, Thiamin Mononitrate [Vitamin B1], Riboflavin [Vitamin B2], Folic Acid), Vegetable Oil (Canola, Cottonseed, Palm, Sunflower and/or **Partially Hydrogenated** Soybean Oil with TBHQ for freshness), Skim Milk Cheese (Skim Milk, Whey Protein, Cheese Cultures, Salt, Enzymes, Annatto Extract for color), Contains Two Percent or less of Milk, Salt, Paprika, Yeast, Paprika Oleoresin for color, Cheese Cultures, Soy Lecithin.

CHEEZY KALE CHIPS

Kale . . . what a great leaf. A deep, dark green that is superrich in nutrients. Kids love kale chips and I know you will too! This kale chip recipe is hands-down the best I have ever tasted. "Dino" kale is my favorite kale to use for making kale chips. It has a slightly sweeter and more delicate taste than curly kale. Its flat leaves resemble dinosaur skin. These flat leaves also make it easier to work with when making chips. Dinosaur kale is also known as lacinato or Tuscan kale.

2 bunches dinosaur kale (aka Tuscan, lacinato, or black kale), cleaned	Not-Cho-Cheeze Sauce (page 32), made without the chile pepper

1. Set up a dehydrator and line the trays with nonstick sheets.

2. Destem the kale and leave in large pieces. Coat with the Not-Cho-Cheeze Sauce. Lay the coated leaves onto the lined trays. Dehydrate at 115°F for 8 hours.

3. Remove the liners and continue to dry another 8 hours. It is no disaster if you put these in overnight and sleep through removing the liners until morning. Remove them when you get around to it, and then continue to dry until your chips are crispy. This is why raw food is great for busy (or forgetful) people.

SERVES 6

Option: For a Kool Ranch Kale Chip, coat your kale with my Home On the Range Dressing (page 12) and follow the same dehydrating directions. Super yum!!!

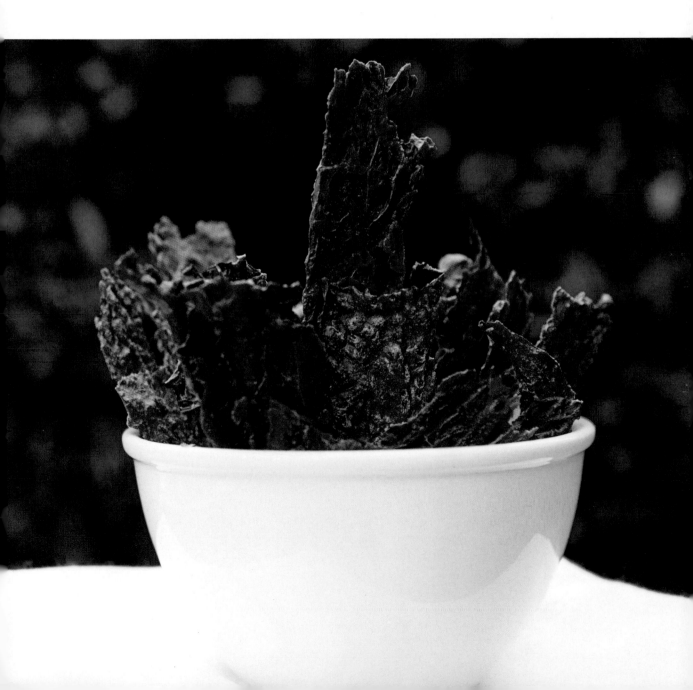

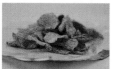

25

LAY'S® KETTLE COOKED SEA SALT & VINEGAR FLAVORED CHIPS

If you want to lose belly fat, put the potato chips down. These are "empty" calories, meaning there is no nutritional value at all. These are simply fat carriers, going right to your belly, hips, and butt. Sitting at a desk and chasing them down with diet sodas will only give you a short-term sense of pleasure. What our bodies truly crave is real food. We crave feeling good all the time.

Just for today . . . do something different.

Ingredients: Potatoes, Vegetable Oil (Sunflower, Canola, and/or Corn Oil), Sea Salt & Vinegar Seasoning (Maltodextrin [Made from Corn], Sea Salt, Vinegar, Buttermilk, Lactose, Sugar, Dextrose, Citric Acid, and Sunflower Oil).

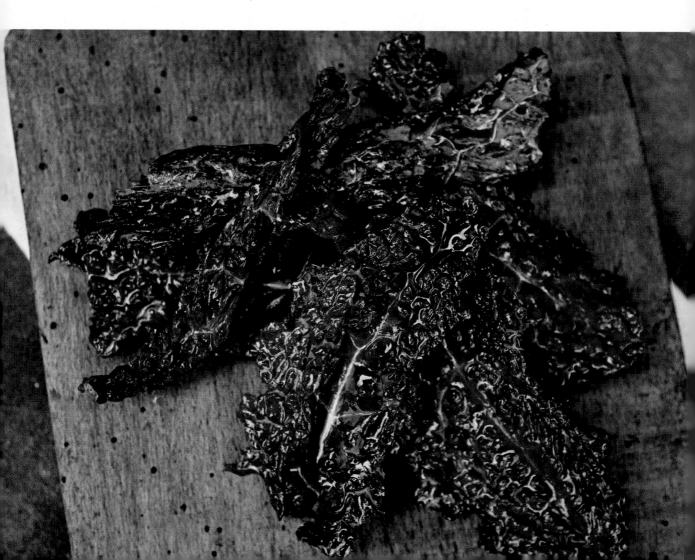

SWEET TANGY KALE CHIPS

When meeting a new family, many times I choose what I think will really wow them, and other times I think of what I am personally hankering for and start by making that recipe first. Your family too will hanker for this perfect combination of a sweet, sour, and salty chip . . . all while eating your greens! Beware, kale chips always bring out the "drator raiders"! This is a term for those little hands that open up the dehydrator and eat half the chips before they are done.

3 bunches dinosaur kale (aka Tuscan, lacinato, or black kale), cleaned

1½ teaspoons sea salt

3 ounces fresh lemon juice

3 ounces olive oil

2 to 3 ounces raw honey, to taste

1. Set up a dehydrator and line the trays with nonstick sheets.

2. Destem the kale and leave in large pieces. Pat dry.

3. In a large bowl, mix together the salt, lemon juice, olive oil, and honey. Add the kale pieces. With your hands, massage the mixture into your kale. Lay out onto the dehydrator trays. Dehydrate at 115°F for 10 hours or until crispy.

SERVES 6

10 REASONS TO EAT YOUR KALE . . .

1. Kale strengthens the immune system, fights bacteria, and wards off viruses.

2. Good news for those who are anemic, kale has more iron than beef, and helps oxygen to get to your blood.

3. Like other dark-green veggies, kale prevents certain types of cancers, such as colon, prostate, and ovarian cancers.

4. The vitamin C content in kale helps relieve stiff joints.

5. The omega-3 fatty acids in kale alleviate asthma, autoimmune disorders, and arthritis.

6. The fiber in kale lowers cholesterol.

7. Vitamin A in kale is great for your eyesight.

8. Per calorie, kale has more calcium than whole milk!

9. Kale is full of fiber and sulfur, both ideal for detoxifying your body and keeping your liver healthy.

10. Kale is hearty and filling. With only 36 calories a cup, kale is a perfect food for weight management.

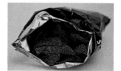

26

DORITOS® SPICY NACHO FLAVORED TORTILLA CHIPS

Monosodium glutamate (MSG) is actually injected into laboratory mice to induce obesity. Why are we eating this stuff? **Artificial flavors:** Companies add "natural" and artificial flavorings to make products taste better. Both are chemically altered and created in a lab. (Homemade foods prepared with fresh ingredients never need such flavorings. Always eat fresh!) **Artificial colors:** Several countries throughout Europe have banned artificial dyes and require any still approved unnatural colorings to display warning labels stating that these artificial dyes may be linked to behavioral issues in children. Doritos could one day be considered child abuse.

No wonder these chips won't decompose. No self-respecting fungus or bacteria will touch this stuff. Keep in mind fungus and bacteria will eat poop.

Ingredients: Corn Whole, Vegetable(s) Oil Contains One or More of the Following (Corn Oil, Soybean(s) Oil or, Sunflower Oil), Maltodextrin, Salt, Cheese Cheddar (Milk Cultured, Salt, Enzyme(s)), Whey, **Monosodium Glutamate**, Buttermilk Solids, Cheese Romano from Cow's Milk (Milk Part Skim Pasteurized Cultured, Salt, Enzyme(s)), Corn Starch, Whey Protein Concentrate, Soybean(s) Oil Partially Hydrogenated, Cottonseed Oil Partially Hydrogenated, Lactose, Disodium Phosphate, Garlic Powder, Dextrose, **Flavor(s) Natural & Artificial**, Onion(s) Powder, Spice(s), **Color(s) Artificial** Includes (Yellow 6 Lake, Red 40 Lake, Yellow 6, Yellow 5, Red 40, Blue 1), Sugar, Citric Acid, Sodium Caseinate, Lactic Acid, Pepper(s) Jalapeno(s) Powder, Disodium Inosinate, Disodium Guanylate, Milk Non-Fat Solids.

JUST A FEW THINGS I LOVE ABOUT NORI . . .

1. Just one sheet of nori has more omega-3 fatty acids than a cup of avocado and more fiber than a cup of spinach!

2. Nori exceeds all land vegetables in protein, vitamins, minerals, and iodine.

3. Nori boosts energy and stamina.

4. Nori enhances your immune, endocrine, digestive, cardiovascular, and nervous systems.

5. Nori excites sexual desires because we have more energy and less pain and stress in the body.

SPICY NORI NACHOS

Why eat sea vegetables? They are jam-packed with minerals, which means they are extremely beneficial for our bodies. Minerals help prevent disease such as high blood pressure, heart disease, osteoporosis, and some cancers. Seaweeds contain all the minerals found in the ocean. These same minerals all happen to be found in our blood.

Not-Cho-Cheeze Sauce (page 32), made without the chile pepper

Optional: red pepper flakes for a little kick
2 packages raw untoasted nori

1. Set up a dehydrator.

2. Make the Not-Cho-Cheeze Sauce and add a sprinkling of red pepper flakes if you'd like.

3. Lay down your nori sheet onto a flat surface and spread a thin layer of Cheeze Sauce on half of the sheet. Fold the other half over. It's like a nori sandwich. Lay the filled nori sheets onto the dehydrator trays. Dehydrate for 8 hours. Once they begin to dry out, you can cut them into triangles with kitchen scissors. Continue to dehydrate for another 8 to 12 hours. When they are crispy, they are done!

Note: When dehydrating nori, always dehydrate alone. Otherwise everything in your dehydrator will have a slight nori taste.

MAKES ABOUT 40 CHIPS

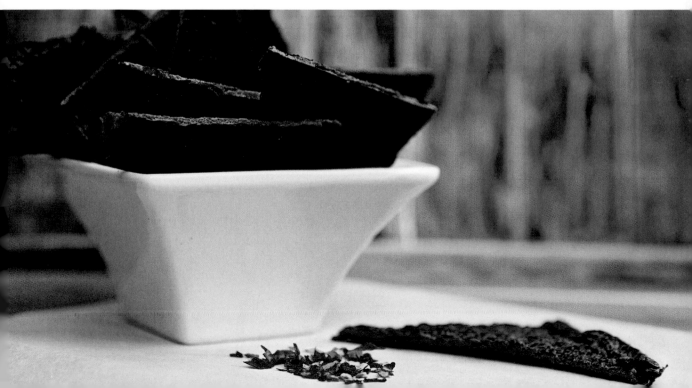

27

BURGER KING® SMALL BASIC ONION RINGS

What's in a BK Onion Ring?

Hydrogenated oils are only one molecule away from being plastic. These oils make it much harder for our hearts to pump blood throughout our systems, which contributes to high blood pressure.

Ingredients: Rehydrated Onion, Bleached Wheat Flour, **Partially Hydrogenated Soybean Oil**, Water, Yellow Corn Flour, Sugar, Contains 2% or less of the following: Gelatinized Wheat Starch, Corn Starch, Calcium Chloride, Modified Food Starch, Methylcellulose, Salt, Fructose, Guar Gum, Sodium Alginate, Yeast, Sodium Bicarbonate, Glucano Delta Lactone, Sodium Tripolyphosphate, Sodium Acid Pyrophosphate, Sodium Aluminum Phosphate, Natural Onion Flavor, Garlic Powder, Hydroxyl Propyl Methylcellulose, Sorbitol.

ONION RINGS

Onion rings are awesome! And these are the easiest things to throw into the dehydrator. They make a great snack but also decorate a meal or a salad beautifully. I use cashews in the coating, which gives the onions that hint of sweetness you find in a traditional onion ring batter. Always choose sweet onions for this recipe. They are going to be mild in flavor and less hot than another type of onion. The nutritional yeast flakes will give your onion rings a salty taste, so it is not necessary to add additional salt.

1 cup raw cashews, ground into a flour
½ cup nutritional yeast flakes (not brewer's yeast—read the product label carefully before you buy)

2 medium sweet onions
Olive oil, just enough to lightly coat the onions

1. Set up a dehydrator.

2. In a small bowl, stir together the cashew flour and yeast flakes.

3. Slice the onions into rings and in a large bowl, coat the onion rings lightly in olive oil.

4. In a third bowl, working with a handful at a time, lightly coat the onion rings with the flour mixture. Working in batches will prevent your coating from clumping.

5. Lay the onion rings onto the dehydrator trays. Dehydrate at 115°F for 10 to 12 hours.

SERVES 12

THE AMAZING ONION!

Besides being very low in calories and tasting really good, onions and the onion relatives (garlic, leeks, chives, scallions, and spring onions) are the top vegetables across the board in preventing cancers. These onion rings are raw, which means all their super powers are still intact!

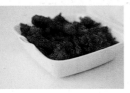

28

LONG JOHN SILVER'S FRIED CLAMS

You are going to be getting a lot of chemically enhanced fried dough when you head to Long John Silver's. In fact, these fried dough "crumblies" are what draws people like sharks to chum. A box of clam strips are 320 calories with 170 calories coming from fat, and that is not the "good" fat.

Ingredients in the fried dough batter: Wheat Flour, Corn Starch, Yellow Corn Flour, Salt, MSG, Spices (Including Paprika), Baking Soda, Garlic Powder, Natural Flavoring.

NOT FRIED, NOT CLAMS

Yes, it's true! These really do taste like fried clams. One calamari-loving family likened them to fried calamari bites. These little snacks rarely make it off the dehydrator trays before they are all eaten up. Follow the same directions for Onion Rings (page 68). This flour mixture will use walnuts, which always give a meatier flavor versus a cashew, which gives things a creamy sweet flavor.

1½ cups walnuts, ground into flour
½ cup nutritional yeast flakes

1 large head cauliflower
Olive oil, just enough to lightly coat the cauliflower

1. Set up a dehydrator.

2. In a small bowl, mix together the walnut flour and nutritional yeast flakes.

3. Cut the cauliflower into pieces the size of a Lego or a Barbie doll shoe. In a large bowl, coat the cauliflower lightly in olive oil.

4. In a third bowl, working with a handful at a time, lightly coat the cauliflower with the flour mixture. Working in batches will prevent your coating from clumping.

5. Lay the cauliflower onto the dehydrator trays. Dehydrate at 115°F for 18 to 24 hours.

SERVES 4

THE WALNUT

If you are not a fan of fish, but want to get your healthy unsaturated fats and omega-3 fatty acids, eat walnuts! Omega-3 fatty acids are excellent for fighting inflammation. Walnuts also contain more antioxidants than any other nut. Antioxidants help protect the body from cellular damage that contributes to cancer, premature aging, and heart disease. If PMS is getting you down, eat a handful of raw walnuts. The magnesium they contain could turn your day right around.

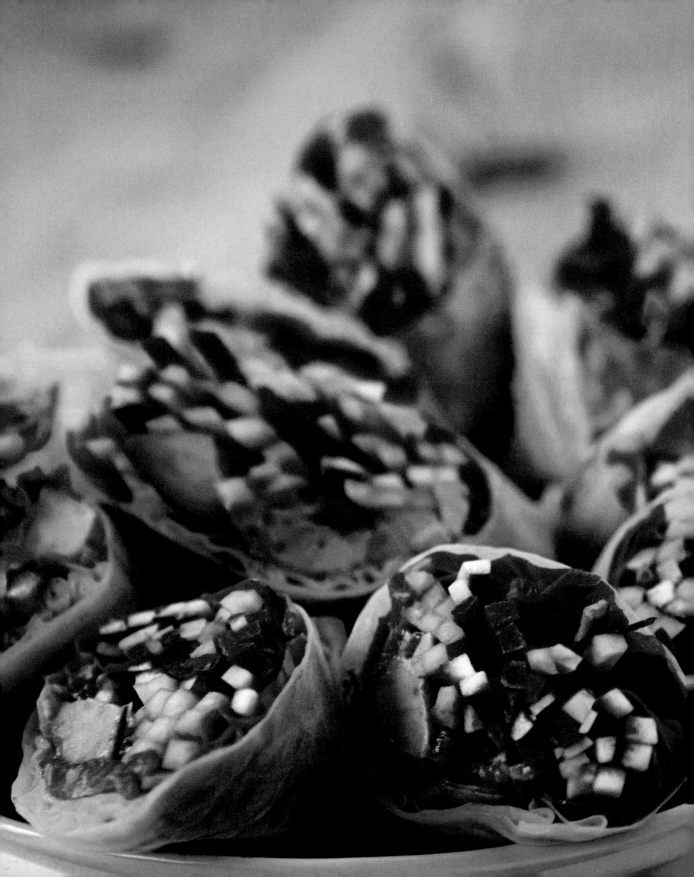

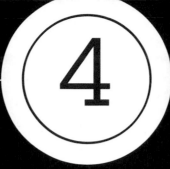

Family Favorites

Broccoli Alfredo

Italian "Pasta"

Raw Pizza

Lasagna

Firehouse Tostadas

Stacy's Guacamole

The Perfect Picnic Burger

Mac & Cheeze

Rainbow Fajitas

China Bowl

Thuy's Pad Thai

Spring Rolls

▪ Always Eat Pretty! ▪

You are about to create the most savory form of art, and these recipes are a great place for you to begin. We've been given such an astounding array of color in our plant kingdom. Let's take full advantage of the rainbow of colors in front of us. Remember, our eyes always eat before our stomachs do, so when creating any dish or salad, I always use at least three colors. Feel free to add more colors, but never fewer than three. I also like to create at least three layers and three textures to any given dish.

Why is three the magic number? I learned this technique of "threes" when decorating, and many use the same philosophy when arranging flowers. In decorating, you always use an odd number of placing things—I like groupings of three.

REINVENTING THE KITCHEN: BRINGING PARENTS AND KIDS TOGETHER

Preventable obesity-related diseases continues to be on the rise, while health officials' forecasts seem to be pretty bleak for our children's future. It has been projected that by 2030, medical costs associated with treating these diseases could increase to $66 billion per year in the United States. We can't afford this. Change is needed.

We need a plan of action. This is not a problem for our government or our schools. Home is where to start. We must do two things: (1) get off processed foods and (2) begin adding in more nutritionally rich RAW plant-based foods.

Parents, start 'em young, by introducing our planet's best foods to your toddlers—vegetables! A green blended smoothie is a perfect first food! Let kids be part of the solution. Shop for food together. Talk about what's in our food. Avoid food ingredients you can't pronounce. Get your kids in the kitchen with you. Play. A kitchen can bring families together if we start early. Let's reinvent the kitchen!

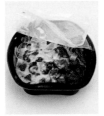

29

WEIGHT WATCHER'S BROCCOLI ALFREDO

Diet foods and sodas are keeping us fat! Many of us are tempted by these low-calorie "fake foods." The numbers do not always tell the whole story. Processed foods are highly acidic, which in turn creates an acidic environment in our bodies. When we are acidic, our bodies will store acidity in fat, making it harder for us to lose excess weight. Lesson: Eat real food.

Ingredients: Alfredo Sauce (Water, Parmesan Cheese [Milk, Cheese Culture, Salt, Enzymes], Skim Milk, Modified Cornstarch, Milk, Potato Maltodextrin, contains less than 2% of Ammonium Chloride, Butter [Cream, Salt], Buttermilk Solids, Calcium Lactate, Calcium Phosphate, Cheddar Cheese Flavor [Milk, Salt, Enzymes, Cultures], Citric Acid, Cream, Dehydrated Cheese [Milk, Cheese Culture, Salt, Enzymes], Lactic Acid, Lactose, Corn Maltodextrin, Mannitol, Natural Flavor, Potassium Chloride, Potassium Citrate, Salt, Sodium Phosphate, Soy Lecithin, Spice, Sunflower Oil, Whey, Whey Protein Concentrate, Xanthan Gum, Yeast Extract), Cooked Enriched Cavatappi Pasta (Water, Enriched Semolina [Durum Wheat Semolina, Niacin, Iron, Thiamine Mononitrate, Riboflavin, Folic Acid], Cooked Chicken White Meat (Chicken White Meat, Water, Isolated Soy Protein, Modified Cornstarch, Chicken Flavor [Dehydrated Chicken Broth, Chicken Powder, Natural Flavor], Sodium Phosphate, Salt, Dehydrated Garlic, Black Pepper, Caramel Coloring, Flavoring [Potassium Chloride, Tricalcium Phosphate, Sunflower Seed Oil, Medium Chain Triglycerides, Acetic Acid, Flavor]), Broccoli.

BROCCOLI ALFREDO

The Broccoli Alfredo is the very first meal I serve when I meet a new family. Why? Because it is so quick and easy, making more time for us all to get acquainted . . . and it tastes amazing! This broccoli dish also goes well alongside Italian "Pasta" (page 77). Broccoli Alfredo turns into a beautiful meal when you add it to a few more vegetable layers. I call this "nesting." First make a fluffy nest of arugula on your plate that has been lightly tossed in olive oil. Inside your arugula nest, add a hand full of julienned zucchini noodles. Lastly, top your first two nests with your Broccoli Alfredo. Garnish with some pine nuts, avocado, and a few sprigs of basil.

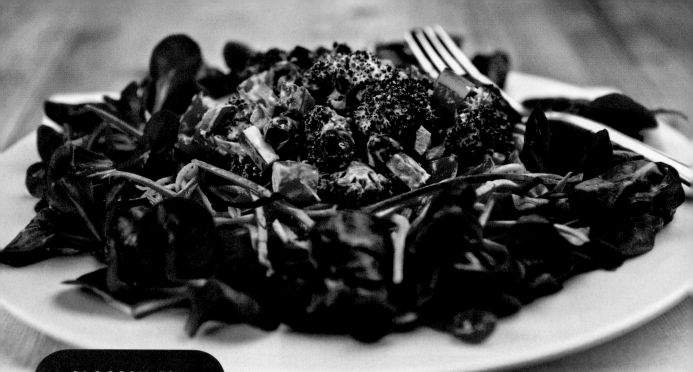

BROCCOLI FOR OUR BONES!

One cup of raw broccoli has 25 calories, 0g fat, and 2g fiber. Broccoli contains high levels of both calcium and vitamin K, both of which are important for bone health and prevention of osteoporosis.

4 to 5 cups bite-size broccoli florets

Basic White Sauce (page 22) to taste (make sure it is a thick creamy consistency for easy coating) or Home on the Range Dressing (page 12)

1 red or yellow bell pepper, diced

½ cup pitted kalamata olives, sliced

Arugula, for serving

Olive oil, for coating

Julienned zucchini noodles

Optional: Pine nuts, avocado, and basil sprigs, for garnish

1. In a large bowl, coat the broccoli florets evenly with the Basic White Sauce. Now add the bell pepper and olives.

2. In a second bowl, toss the arugula with a little olive oil. Make a nest of arugula on a plate. Top that with a smaller nest of zucchini noodles. Spoon the broccoli mixture on top. Garnish with some pine nuts, avocado, and a few sprigs of basil if desired. Serve additional sauce on the side.

SERVES 6

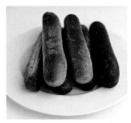

30

OLIVE GARDEN'S FIVE-CHEESE ZITI AL FORNO

Most Italian pasta meals are also served with a lot of bread. There are absolutely no nutritional deficiencies that result from eliminating bread from one's diet. It is "filler," and if you fill up on bread, you miss out on eating the most nutritionally *rich* foods on our planet—vegetables.

Three breadsticks (the bread basket is endless, but we will stop at three): 420 calories, 6g fat, 78g carbohydrates. The small lunch-size entree of baked ziti (double the numbers for the dinner portion): 528 calories, 22g fat, 60g carbohydrates.

ITALIAN "PASTA"

I pair two types of noodles—a raw zucchini noodle and a cooked spaghetti squash noodle—with my marinara sauce. This threesome comes together beautifully in color, flavor, and texture. The perfect complement to this "pasta" meal is the creamy Broccoli Alfredo (page 75), served as a side dish. The Onion Rings (page 68) complete the meal as a perfect garnish!

1 medium spaghetti squash (see Note), cooked	Tyrannosaurus Red Sauce (page 34)
6 to 8 zucchinis	

1. Preheat the oven to 375°F.

2. Halve the spaghetti squash lengthwise or in quarters. You don't want to cut it up too small unless you want short strands. Scrape out the seeds and stringy pulp as you would with any squash or pumpkin. Place onto a baking sheet cut side down and bake until fork-tender, 30 to 40 minutes. (As an alternative, you can cook the squash in boiling water for about 20 minutes.) Scrape out the cooked squash with a fork. It should fall out easily.

3. Spaghetti squash has a very mild sweet flavor, thus it serves nicely with all the other flavors on your plate. Add a little sea salt and a bit of unrefined coconut oil, to taste, before serving. The cooked spaghetti squash is going to add some warmth and comfort to this Italian pasta dinner.

4. Use your julienne peeler to transform raw zucchini into these amazing noodles, using the outer sides of the zucchinis but not the inner seedy core. Cut the noodles into 2-inch pieces for easier eating. Since the seedy part of the zucchini will not hold up as a noodle, save it and add to Sunny Slope Farm Soup (page 108).

5. On each plate, serve ½ to 1 cup each zucchini noodles and spaghetti squash noodles side by side. Top the noodles with ¼ to ½ cup Tyrannosaurus Red Sauce.

Note: Spaghetti squash is also a good alternative to pasta. The cooked squash flesh shreds into threads like thin spaghetti, hence its name. On average, a spaghetti squash measures about 12 inches in length and about 6 inches in diameter. The squash should be an even light yellow color and firm with no bruises. Store whole at room temperature up to 3 weeks. Spaghetti squash is available year-round with peak season in Fall.

SERVES 8 TO 10

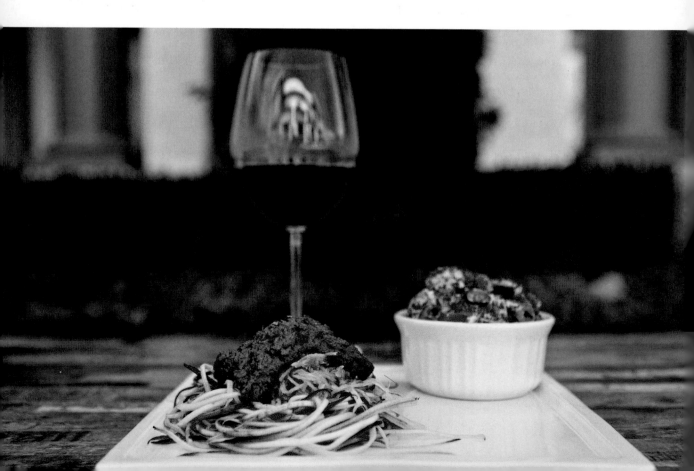

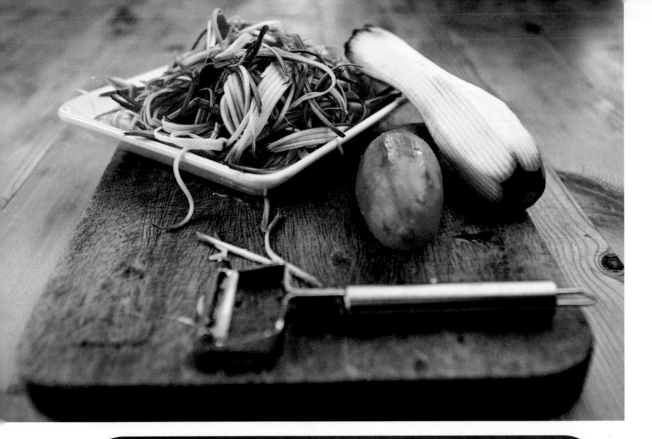

ZUCCHINI "PASTA" NOODLES

If you are searching for a healthy and low-carbohydrate pasta alternative, try substituting raw zucchini noodles in your favorite pasta dishes. Zucchini and summer squash are mild vegetables, so they complement a lot of different meals, as they take on the flavors of the dish, whether Asian or Italian. Cut into thin noodle strips using a julienne vegetable peeler.

High in fiber, water, vitamin A, vitamin C, and potassium, zucchini offers an abundance of nutrients to support your health. The water and fiber in this tender summer squash will help manage your weight by providing low-calorie volume. One cup of zucchini noodles only has 20 calories. Its vitamins and minerals promote the health of your heart, eyes, skin, and lungs, while boosting your immune system. The most nutrient-rich part of this vegetable is the dark green skin.

Yellow squash is another highly nutritious piece of summer goodness. Free radicals are known to cause skin cancer, premature aging of the skin, and sun damage. Yellow squash is full of anti-oxidants, known for fighting these free radicals. Kinda makes you crave some yellow squash this summer!

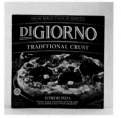

31

DIGIORNO SUPREME PIZZA FOR ONE, TRADITIONAL CRUST

Q: How do you make mechanically separated chicken taste good?

A: Mix in textured soy protein, food coloring, laboratory created pork flavor, pork fat, sugar, salt, lots of stuff I can't pronounce, and the oh-so-very-important taste enhancer, MSG, disguised as autolyzed yeast extract (just one of this chemical's pseudonyms).

Ingredients: Enriched Wheat Flour (Wheat Flour, Niacin, Reduced Iron, Thiamine Mononitrate, Riboflavin, Folic Acid), Water, Shredded Low-Moisture Part-Skim Mozzarella Cheese (Part-Skim Milk, Cheese Culture, Salt, Enzymes), Cooked Seasoned Pizza Topping (Pork, Water, Mechanically Separated Chicken, Textured Vegetable Protein [Soy Protein Concentrate, Caramel Color], Spices, Salt, Sugar, Sodium Phosphate, Paprika, Pork Flavor [Modified Corn Starch, Pork Fat, Natural Flavors, Pork Stock, Gelatin, Autolyzed Yeast Extract, Sodium Phosphate, Thiamine Hydrochloride, Sunflower Oil, Propyl Gallate], Caramel Color, Spice Extractives, BHA, BHT, Citric Acid, Cooked in Pork Fat or Beef Fat or Vegetable Oil), Tomato Paste, Pepperoni Made with Pork, Chicken and Beef (Pork, **Mechanically Separated Chicken**, Beef, Salt, contains 2% or less of Pork Stock, Spices, Dextrose, Lactic Acid Starter Culture, Paprika, Natural Smoke Flavor, Oleoresin Paprika, Sodium Ascorbate, Sodium Nitrite, Flavoring, BHA, BHT, Citric Acid), Green Bell Peppers, Red Bell Peppers, Sugar, contains less than 2% of Wheat Gluten, Onions, Black Olives, Vegetable Oil (Soybean Oil and/or Corn Oil), White Corn Meal, Salt, Yellow Corn Meal, Baking Powder (Baking Soda, Sodium Aluminum Phosphate), Yeast, Sodium Stearoyl Lactylate, DATEM, Flavor, Spice, Dried Garlic, Ascorbic Acid.

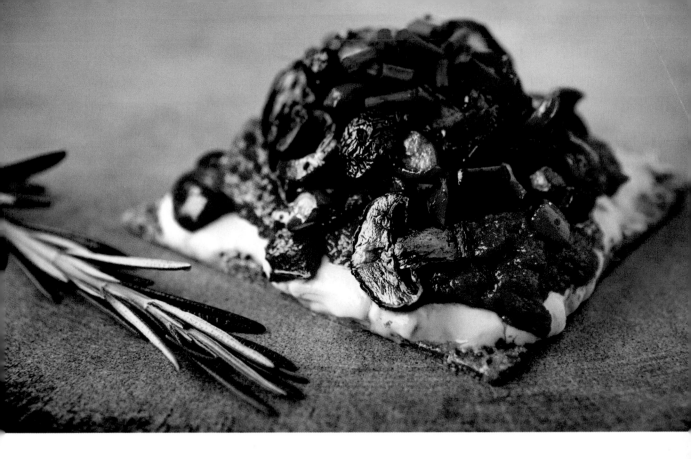

RAW PIZZAS

Very often after serving the Italian "Pasta" (page 77) with Broccoli Alfredo (page 75), I will have leftover Tyrannosaurus Red Sauce (page 34) and Basic White Sauce (page 22). What better way to utilize leftovers than on a pizza!

CHEEZE: ¾ cup Basic White Sauce (page 22), made with ⅔ cup water

CRUST: Seeds of Change (page 56) or Flagels (page 46)

TOPPING: Marinated Veggie Topping (page 82)

SAUCE: ¾ cup Tyrannosaurus Red Sauce (page 34) or Better Than Ketchup (page 16)

1. Make the cheeze sauce a day ahead and chill. It will thicken to cheese consistency as it chills.

2. Make the marinated veggies the day before.

FAMILY FAVORITES

■ 81 ■

3. Make the crusts, cutting the Seeds of Change into sandwich bread–size squares or triangles.

4. For each individual pizza crust, layer on 2 tablespoons cheeze (note that the cheeze layer comes first, which keeps your crust from possibly getting soggy) and top with 2 tablespoons pizza sauce. Top with ⅓ to ¼ cup marinated veggie topping. Garnish with a sprig of basil.

MAKES 6 MINI PIZZAS

MARINATED VEGGIE TOPPING

1 cup sliced mushrooms

1 cup chopped zucchini

1 cup chopped red bell pepper

Super Simple Marinade (page 36)

1. In a large bowl, toss the mushrooms, zucchini, and bell pepper with the marinade.

2. Marinate overnight.

3. Set up a dehydrator and line the trays with nonstick sheets. Spread the vegetables on the trays and dehydrate at 115°F for 3 hours.

MAKES ENOUGH TO TOP 6 MINI PIZZAS

WHAT ARE THE SIDE EFFECTS OF NOT GETTING ENOUGH RAW VEGETABLES?

CONSTIPATION is the most common form of digestive trouble affecting everyone from our toddlers to our elderly. Raw vegetables are an excellent source of fiber, which keeps us regular.

VITAMIN AND MINERAL DEFICIENCY. Depending on what vitamins and minerals we are lacking, we could run into any number of weaknesses in our body. Our bodies are strengthened, and function at peak performance, when we eat plenty of raw vegetables.

WEIGHT GAIN. If you are not getting enough calories from raw vegetables, those calories are more than likely coming from other sources, like fat and carbohydrates. If you eat more raw vegetables, you will not be indulging in unhealthier food choices that lead to excess weight gain.

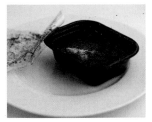

32

STOUFFER'S LASAGNA

Americans are not getting enough raw vegetables. Our breakfast, lunch, and dinner plates continue to be made up of mostly breads, meats, and cheeses. A hefty lasagna dish is a prime example, and that side salad bathed in dressing, croutons, and cheese is just not gonna cut it.

Ingredients: Tomato Puree (Water Tomato Paste), Blanched Macaroni Product (Water, Semolina) Part Skim Mozzarella Cheese and Modified Cornstarch (Part-Skim Mozzarella Cheese [Pasteurized Milk, Salt, Cultures, Enzymes], Modified Cornstarch, Nonfat Milk, Flavors), Beef, Water, Dry Curd Cottage Cheese (Cultured Skim Milk, Enzymes), 2% or less of Modified Cornstarch, Salt, Bleached Wheat Flour, Dehydrated Onions, Sugar, Spices, Seasoning (Soy Sauce [Water, Soybean, Wheat, Salt], Autolyzed Yeast Extract, Dextrose, Soybean Oil), Dehydrated Garlic, Yeast Extract, Carrageenan. Warning: Contains milk, soy, wheat ingredients.

LASAGNA

This is not your typical raw lasagna found in raw food restaurants around the country. It is a lovely warm comfort food.

1 cup Basic White Sauce (page 22), made with ⅔ cup water

Marinated Veggie Topping (page 82)

8 medium zucchinis

Olive oil, for coating

2 cups chopped fresh spinach

1½ cups of Tyrannosaurus Red Sauce (page 34)

½ cup sliced tomatoes or sliced grape tomatoes.

10 fresh basil leaves

Arugula, for serving

Fresh lemon juice, for coating

Pine nuts, for garnish

1. Make the Basic White Sauce a day ahead and chill so it will thicken up. Start the marinated veggies the day before.

2. Set up a dehydrator.

3. Peel the zucchinis with a flat-bladed "potato" peeler. (Leave behind the seedy inner part of the zucchini and save for a nice Sunny Slope Farm Soup, page 108.) This will give you a lot of very thin flat strips. Cut into approximately 2-inch strips

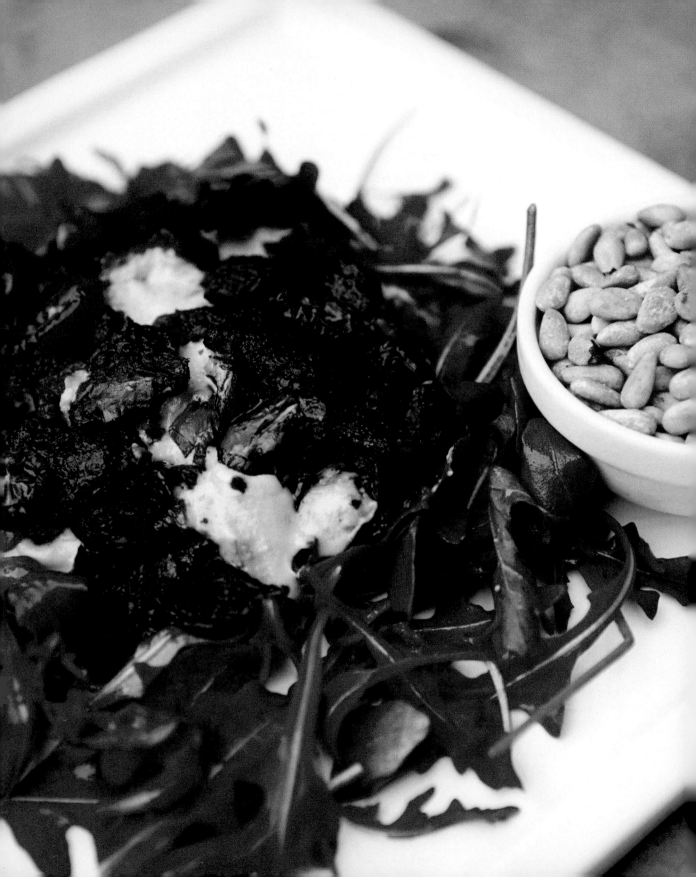

(no perfection necessary). This makes for easier eating. Coat these 2-inch zucchini strips with olive oil. Lay out on trays and dehydrate at 115°F overnight or until dried like a chip. This step will ensure you don't end up with lasagna floating in water.

4. In an 11 x 7-inch glass baking dish, build your lasagna layers. Make a layer of half the dried zucchini, half of the spinach, half of the Basic White Sauce, half of the marinated veggies, and ¾ cup of the Tyrannosaurus Red Sauce. (Note: Place dollops of the Basic White Sauce and the Tyrannosaurus Red Sauce. Trying to spread these sauces into your layers is both time-consuming and not necessary.)

5. Repeat the layers. Top the lasagna with sliced tomatoes and basil leaves. Put the lasagna in the bottom of the dehydrator for 1 hour at 145°F, turn down the heat to 115°F for an additional 1 to 2 hours. You will have a lasagna that will be warm and will have that baked appearance we love about this favorite comfort food.

6. Toss some arugula with a little lemon juice and olive oil. Serve the lasagna on a bed of the dressed arugula. Sprinkle with a few pine nuts.

SERVES 8

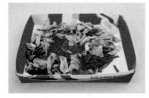

33

TACO BELL TOSTADA (THE BEANS)

What's TBHQ? Tertiary butylhydroquinone (TBHQ) is a "harmless additive"—namely, a form of butane (i.e., lighter fluid). The FDA will only allow processors to use it sparingly in our food. You would have to eat a lot of beans before side effects like nausea, vomiting, delirium, and/or ringing in the ears set in before you collapse. Don't worry, you will never eat that many beans. Thank you, FDA, for setting a butane limit on our food.

Ingredients: pinto beans, soy oil (with **TBHQ** and citric acid to protect flavor), salt.

FIREHOUSE TOSTADAS

I love to feed our firemen. They live days away from their families each week, while serving their community and putting themselves in dangerous situations to save lives. Firemen must be in peak physical condition, and this is why they need to be fed the most powerful foods on the planet. Raw plant-based foods are for superheroes!

<table>
<tr><td>15 Tostadas (page 58)</td><td>2 cups chopped tomatoes</td></tr>
<tr><td>Stacy's Guacamole (page 88)</td><td>Basic White Sauce (page 22)</td></tr>
<tr><td>3 cups chopped romaine lettuce</td><td></td></tr>
</table>

Top each tostada with a plentiful amount of guacamole and top with chopped lettuce and tomato. Drizzle with Basic White Sauce as your sour cream. You may need to add some additional water to this sauce in order to get a sour cream consistency.

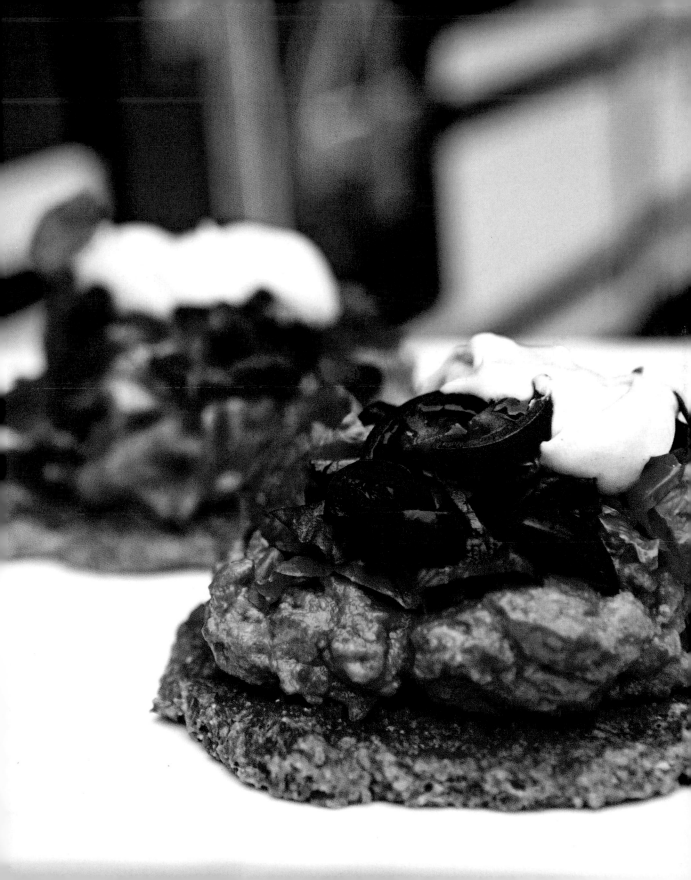

34

DEAN'S GUACAMOLE

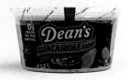

Holy guacamole . . . where are the avocados, Dean? Instead of using avocados, Dean's has cut the cost ($2.00 for 12 ounces) on this "guacamole"-flavored dip by combining fillers, chemicals, modified food starch, plenty of food coloring, and other stuff I can't pronounce.

Today we live in a culture that emphasizes cheap food. The problem is, if we cheap out on our food, we in turn pay more on the other end for health care trying to fix the damage we've done to our bodies. Just for today . . . eat a real avocado ($2.00).

Ingredients: Skim Milk, Soybean Oil, Tomatoes, Water, Coconut Oil, contains less than 2% of Avocado, Whole Egg, Onion*, Salt, Distilled Vinegar, Egg Yolks, Sugar, Nonfat Dry Milk, Whey (Milk), Lactic Acid, Sodium Caseinate (Milk), Isolated Soy Protein, Tomato Juice, Vegetable Mono & Diglycerides, Spices, Sodium Benzoate and Potassium Sorbate (to preserve freshness), Gelatin, Corn Starch, Guar Gum, Cellulose Gel & Cellulose Gum, Lemon Juice Concentrate, Locust Bean Gum, Disodium, Phosphate, Gum Arabic, Xanthan Gum, Cilantro,* Natural Flavors, Extractive Of Paprika, Citric Acid, Ascorbic Acid, Blue 1, Red 40, Yellow 5, Yellow 6.

STACY'S GUACAMOLE

It has been said that avocado is the "gateway" to raw food. This is because it is rich, creamy, full of nutritional benefits, and very, very satisfying. So if you are trying to transition off of a heavy cooked diet, reach for an avocado! Slice some zucchini into little rounds for a quick and easy zucchini chip.

5 large avocados

3 tablespoons fresh lemon juice (this is what makes it my version. I love LEMON!)

3 garlic cloves, minced

½ teaspoon salt, or to taste

1½ cups tomatoes, diced

½ small red onion, diced

In a bowl, mash the avocado, lemon juice, garlic, and salt with your hands. Add the tomatoes and onions.

SERVES 15

* Dehydrated

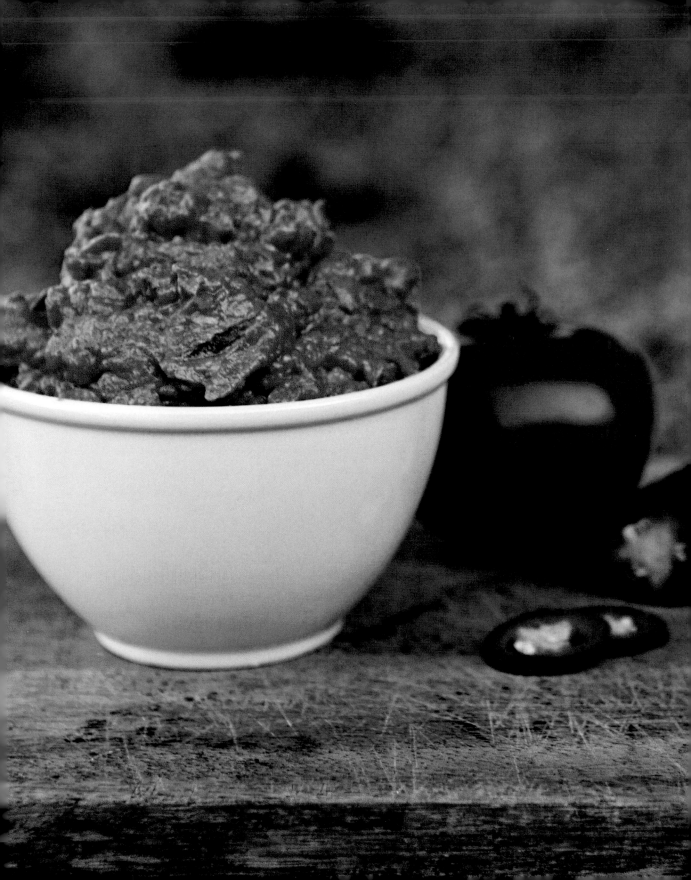

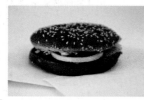

35

THE BURGER

As Americans get bigger, so do their burgers. Years ago, a typical burger would only cost you around 300 calories. Nowadays, burgers range anywhere from 700 calories to 2,000 calories, not to mention all the fat and sodium included.

Burger King Whopper with Cheese: 760 calories, 47g fat, 16g saturated fat, 1,410mg sodium

Chili's Southern Smokehouse Burger: 1,610 calories, 96g fat, 31g saturated fat, 4,530mg sodium

Cheesecake Factory's Ranch House Burger: This burger weighs in at 1,890 calories (fat grams not listed), 48g saturated fat, 2,830 sodium

~~~

THE PERFECT PICNIC BURGER

I think I was the only kid who never liked burgers growing up, so when I was asked to re-create one, I was less than thrilled. Much to my surprise, this burger has become a huge hit with families, and me as well! The Perfect Picnic Burger is filling, full of flavor, and absolutely perfect for picnic packing!

1 cup walnuts	1 Medjool date, pitted
1 cup pumpkin seeds	2 tablespoons tamari
1 cup chopped mushrooms	2 small garlic cloves
½ cup chopped carrots	2 tablespoons olive oil
⅓ cup chopped red bell pepper/	3 tablespoons Italian herb seasoning
⅓ cup oil-packed sun-dried tomatoes, drained	*Optional:* ½ jalapeño pepper (test the heat of your pepper and adjust to taste)

1. In a food processor, combine all the ingredients and process until a sticky consistency. If your mixture is too wet, simply add a bit more walnuts and/or pumpkin seeds. Scoop out ¼ cup and shape into patties. (Or make half-size patties for sliders.)

2. Set up a dehydrator and leave the trays unlined. Place the burgers on the trays and dehydrate for 12 to 18 hours.

MAKES 10 BURGERS OR 20 SLIDERS

BUILDING THE PERFECT PICNIC BURGER

Use butter lettuce instead of a bun, and top with slices of tomato, avocado, red onion, and raw sauerkraut (there are some great raw krauts popping up in grocery stores around our country). Try topping with my Better Than Ketchup (page 16).

One Perfect Picnic Burger with all the fixin's: 234 calories, 18g fat, 11g carbohydrates, 4.9g sugar, 7.9g protein.

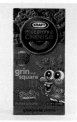

36

KRAFT MACARONI & CHEESE

Quick-cooking noodles in shapes of fun cartoon characters topped with bright orange cheese reminds us of when we were kids. It's time for us to grow up and stop eating like eight-year-olds. In fact, even *our* eight-year-olds should not be eating this stuff.

Do you really want to eat a "cheese" that is colored by dyes and has been sitting in a boxed powder form for months?

Ingredients: Wheat Flour which contains B Vitamins, Niacin, Thiamine, Mono Nitrate, Folic Acid, Riboflavin, Iron in the form of Ferrous Sulfate, Whey (Milk Protein), Milk Protein Concentrate, Milk, Milk Fat, Cheese Culture, Salt, Sodium Tripolyphosphate, Sodium Phosphate, Calcium Phosphate, **Yellow 5, Yellow 6**, Citric Acid, Lactic Acid, and Enzymes.

MAC & CHEEZE

This raw Mac & Cheeze pairs well alongside The Perfect Picnic Burger (page 90), tops a salad nicely, or can simply be enjoyed alone for a kid's quick snack. For making the little half circle macaroni shapes, you will need a special spiral vegetable slicer. The overall best one on the market is World Cuisine Tri-Blade Plastic Vegetable Slicer. I love how easy I can zip right through a squash, creating a big bowl of "noodles." Plus, cleanup is easy and the price of this slicer is around $30. For a great entrée, serve Mac & Cheeze on top a bed of mixed baby greens. Garnish with sliced tomatoes, avocado, kalamata olives, and a little fresh dill.

4 large yellow summer squash

Not-Cho-Cheeze Sauce (page 32), made without the chile pepper

1. Using your vegetable slicer, follow the manufacturer's directions for making noodles out of your yellow summer squash. Cut the long curly noodle strands into little half-circle macaroni shapes.

2. Right before serving, toss the noodles with desired amount of Not-Cho-Cheeze Sauce.

SERVES 4

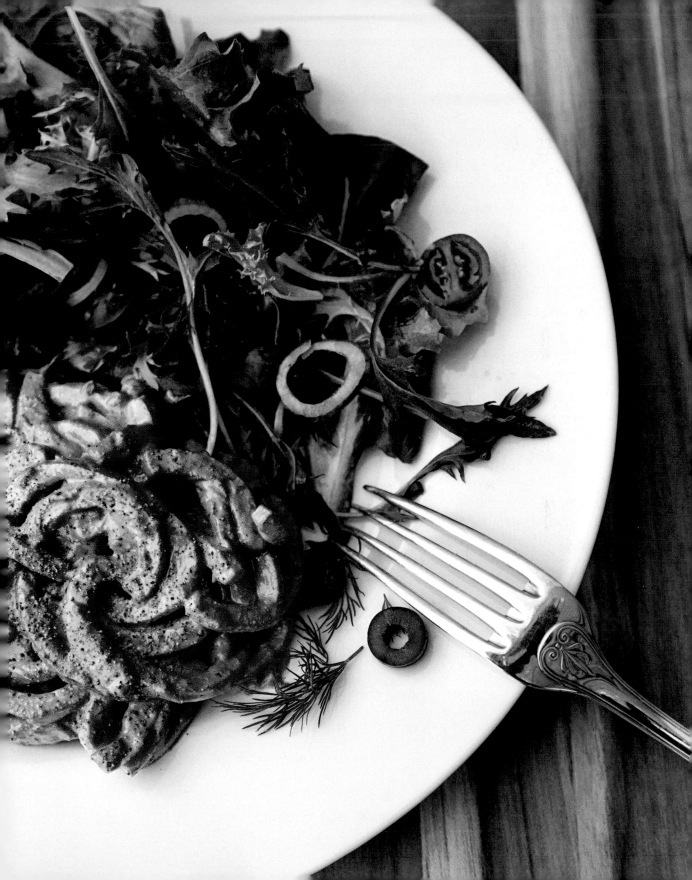

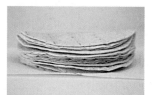

37

THE TORTILLA

Let's talk tortillas (I grew up in South Texas, so I know my tortillas!). Nutritionally speaking, tortillas are "filler food." Bread serves no purpose nutritionally; it is only for filling up and keeping weight on. There are absolutely no vitamin or mineral deficiencies that are caused by eliminating bread. If you want to lose excess weight, snub the tortillas!

RAINBOW FAJITAS

These vegetable fajitas are extremely light and tasty. It's worth investing in a dehydrator for this recipe alone—the marinated/dehydrated vegetables are amazing! I use 6 cups of vegetables in a variety of colors to create an appetizingly colorful plate. Feel free to create your own combination of vegetables, using at least three different colors. Remember, we eat with our *eyes* first.

2 cups sliced portobello mushrooms
1 cup diced red bell pepper
1 cup diced yellow bell pepper
1½ cups sliced zucchini
½ cup sliced red onion

½ cup Super Simple Marinade (page 36)
12 large butter lettuce leaves,
or romaine lettuce leaves
1 cup raw corn, sliced off the cob, for a sweet-flavored garnish
Basic White Sauce (page 22)

1. In a large bowl, toss the vegetables with the Super Simple Marinade and marinate overnight.

2. Set up a dehydrator and line the trays with nonstick sheets. Dehydrate at 115°F for 3 hours.

3. Assemble the fajitas by filling butter lettuce leaves with your fajita filling. Top each fajita with Basic White Sauce, which will serve as your sour cream. Garnish with raw sweet corn.

SERVES 4

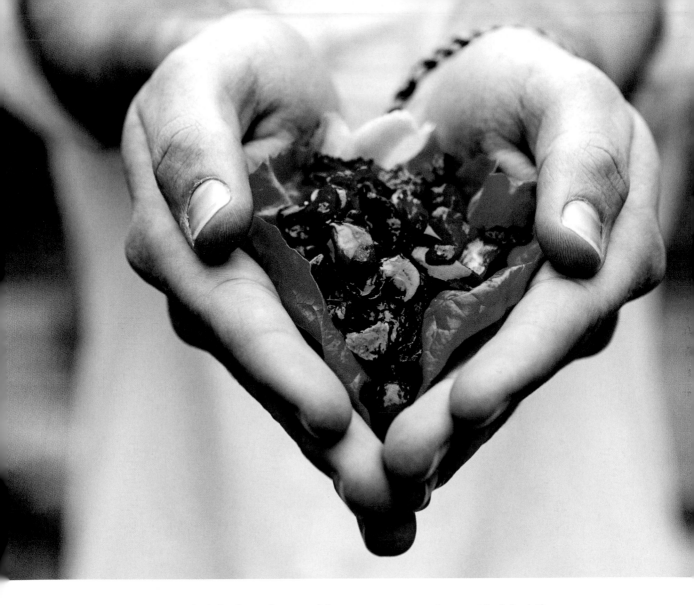

These marinated, dehydrated vegetables may appear to be sautéed, but they are truly raw. Why should we eat all these raw vegetables? Cooking your vegetables destroys digestion-enhancing enzymes, and eating your vegetables raw helps prevent and reverse disease. Raw vegetables are also a wonderful source of vitamins A, C, E, B-complex vitamins, potassium, and calcium. Raw vegetables are super rich in antioxidants and fiber. Because raw vegetables are high in water content, they fill you up, making them a great choice for weight loss.

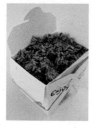

38

CHINESE-AMERICAN FRIED RICE

Flavor enhancers, like Monosodium glutamate, high levels of sodium, and sugar-filled sauces may elevate blood sugar and blood pressure and contribute to cancer, degenerative disorders, weight gain, and heart disease. This is scary stuff!

1 cup of Chinese takeout fried rice: 440 calories, 60g fat, 96g carbohydrates, 4g sugar, 12g protein

CHINA BOWL

Chinese takeout and buffets are about as Chinese as apple pie. While American Chinese food typically treats vegetables as a side dish, the traditional cuisine of China emphasizes vegetables. There is nothing typical or traditional about my China Bowl recipe, but I guarantee we are putting the emphasis on *veggies*! My favorite sauces for this dish are Susie's Spicy Curry Sauce (page 29) and Not Peanut Sauce (page 20).

1 cup sliced mushrooms	½ cup Super Simple Marinade (page 36)
1 cup broccoli florets	1 small head cauliflower
1 cup diced red bell pepper	¼ cup (or less) chopped fresh parsley
1 cup shredded carrots	1 tablespoon olive oil
1 cup sliced zucchini	Salt
1 cup sliced pea pods	

1. In a large bowl, combine the mushrooms, broccoli, bell pepper, carrots, zucchini, and pea pods. Add the Super Simple Marinade, toss to coat, and marinate overnight.

2. Set up a dehydrator and line the trays with nonstick sheets. Arrange the vegetables on the tray and dehydrate at 115°F for 3 hours.

3. Cut the cauliflower into uniform pieces that will fit into the feed tube of a food processor. Fit the processor with the grating blade and shred the cauliflower, creating cauliflower "rice."

4. Pour the shredded cauliflower into a bowl and mix with the parsley, olive oil, and salt to taste.

5. Serve the dehydrated "stir-fry" vegetables on top of the cauliflower "rice."

MAKES 3 TO 4 CUPS

CAULIFLOWER is part of the cruciferous family, along with broccoli, Brussels sprouts, arugula, and kale, to name just a few. Many people are surprised to find out that in preventing cancers, your top vegetables to eat, across the board, come from the cruciferous family. Heat however, destroys the delicate molecules in these vegetables that prevent cancers. For maximum benefits, eat raw, not cooked.

Note: If you have a thyroid condition and have been advised to avoid cruciferous vegetables, there is good news for you. You can still get all the cell protective properties of cruciferous vegetables by consuming broccoli sprouts. This is because the broccoli sprout contains a huge amount of sulforaphane (this is the good stuff) without the goitrogenic substance that people with thyroid conditions want to avoid.

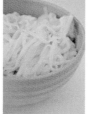

39

PAD THAI NOODLES

Traditional Pad Thai consists of a big bowl of white rice noodles. White rice stores well, takes very little time to prepare, and is inexpensive. White rice will fill people up—and keep weight on as well.

Rice is mostly made up of carbohydrates, which are broken down into sugar and stored in our bodies as fat. When the body needs energy, these fats convert back into sugar for use. But if the body never requires this energy, the fat stays right where it is. So unless you are a marathon runner, rice will contribute to weight gain.

Try switching out these rice noodles with my raw vegetable noodles!

Cooked white rice noodles (per cup): 160 calories, 40g carbohydrates, .08g protein vs.

Raw green papaya noodles (per cup): 55 calories, 14g carbohydrates, 1 gram protein

THUY'S PAD THAI

A green papaya is featured in both traditional and contemporary Vietnamese dishes from spring rolls and salads to main dishes. Unlike the typical sweet tasting, orange papaya you might be familiar with, the inside of the green papaya is white. It is not sweet and, when cut with a julienne peeler, will turn into the most beautiful "noodles" that will hold up in a dressing. Choose a firm, dark-green papaya. I am so happy to have a little Asian market right next to me when I am home in New York. I often carry green papayas in my luggage when I travel to families so that I can share this amazing fruit! One medium papaya will give you 8 cups of noodles. If you simply cannot find a green papaya in your area, don't fret. You can just use all zucchini, yellow squash, and carrots as your noodles. Squash does not hold up in dressings like the hearty green papaya, so dress your noodles right before serving.

RAW GREEN PAPAYA

This is one of the most healing and easily digested fruits. Green papaya is a rejuvenating food choice for all. It is supercharged with vital nutrients including magnesium, potassium, vitamins A, C, B, and E. Green papaya provides plenty of raw live enzymes for improving digestion, which is vital for our bodies to assimilate nutrients, heal, and thrive! Green papaya is ideal for anyone with digestive disorders or low stomach acid. It is also an excellent source of fiber, preventing colon cancer.

6 to 8 cups julienned green papaya

1 large zucchini, cut into julienne noodles (see Note)

1 large carrot, cut into julienne noodles

Not Peanut Sauce (page 20) or Susie's Spicy Curry Sauce (page 29)

1 cup grape tomatoes, halved

1 avocado, sliced

½ cup raw cashews

1 cup tiny sprouted greens, like micro greens, onion sprouts, or arugula sprouts

1. In a large bowl, combine all the vegetable noodles. Right before serving, toss the noodles with your choice of sauce.

2. Pile a heaping cup of noodles on a plate or in a bowl. Garnish with the tomatoes, avocado, and cashews. Top with micro greens.

SERVES 8

Note: When peeling your zucchini for noodles, use the outer portions for noodles and save the seedier inner part for a pot of Sunny Slope Farm Soup (page 108). This outer skin of your squash is the most nutritious part and best eaten raw!

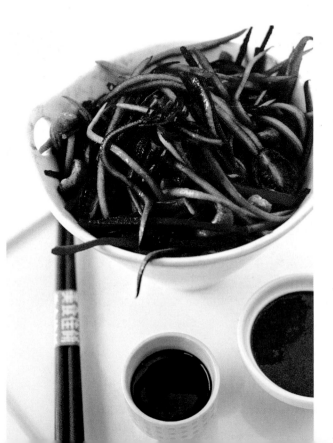

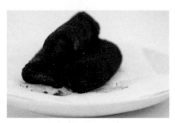

40

EGG ROLLS/SPRING ROLLS

There are several variations of the egg roll. Some people call them egg rolls, some people call them spring rolls—the two terms are often interchangeable. Egg rolls are wrapped in a heavy pastry, while spring rolls are wrapped in a paper-thin, more delicate wrap. Both are typically deep-fried.

COOKING WITH OILS

When oil is heated to temperatures suitable for frying, carcinogens are formed. These carcinogenic compounds increase the risk of cancer. Skip the frying and, when cooking, use coconut oil. All oils turn toxic when heated—except for coconut oil.

COCONUT OIL IS GOOD FOR THE WHOLE FAMILY!

1. Boosts the thyroid.

2. Improves heart health.

3. Supports the immune system.

4. Increases metabolism.

5. Promotes weight loss and keeps us lean

6. When applied topically, coconut oil's regenerative properties act as the best anti-aging skin cream.

7. Coconut oil makes a superb diaper rash cream because of its antibacterial properties.

SPRING ROLLS

In China, spring rolls are closely associated with a spring festival celebrating new growth. How appropriate to share with my families as they venture into a new way of viewing food. Spring rolls are really great for incorporating more raw vegetables into a family's diet. Even kids who won't touch a salad will eat spring rolls! Plus they are fun to make together.

Spring rolls are a large variety of filled, rolled appetizers. The name is a literal translation of the Chinese *chūn juǎn* (春卷, "spring roll") found in East Asian and Southeast Asian cuisine. The kind of wrapper, fillings, and cooking technique used, as well as the name, vary considerably within this large area.

Try an assortment of vegetables like romaine, avocado, and red bell pepper; and julienne-cut vegetables like carrots, zucchini, and yellow summer squash. You will need your handy julienne peeler for this recipe. Serve spring rolls with a side of Not Peanut Sauce (page 20).

1 avocado, sliced	1 yellow summer squash, cut into julienne noodles
½ red bell pepper, cut into strips	Super Simple Marinade (page 36)
1 carrot, cut into julienne noodles	8 romaine lettuce leaves
1 zucchini, cut into julienne noodles	8 rice paper wrappers (8½-inch diameter), sold at most Asian markets and many grocery stores

Cut and slice all vegetables. Right before rolling your spring rolls, toss the julienned vegetable noodles in the Super Simple Marinade and line the rice-paper wrapper with a romaine lettuce leaf. Now we can begin rolling!

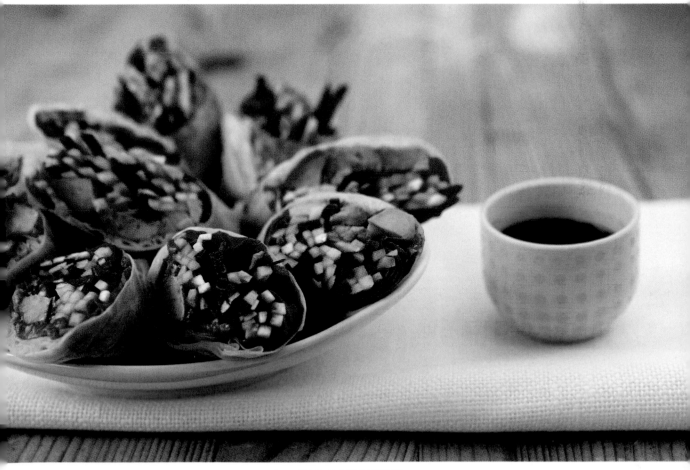

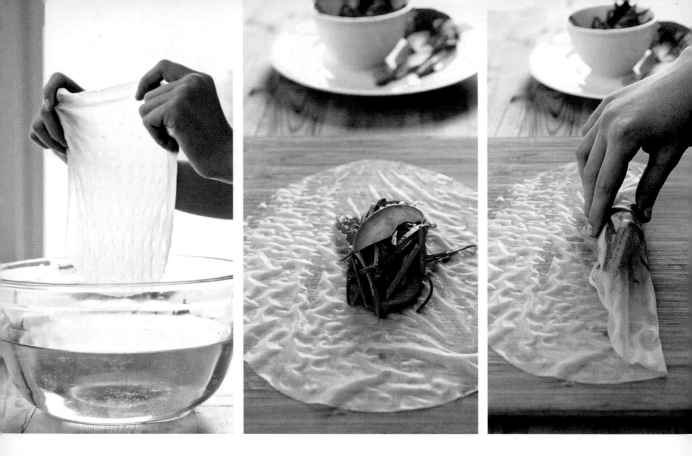

▪ How to Wrap a Spring Roll ▪

If you have never wrapped spring rolls before, it will take a little patience and some practice. The rice paper wrappers are very thin and fragile, so expect to tear a few wrappers at first. This is okay. You can always double-wrap them. Double-wrapping is great for beginners. Another bit of advice: Don't overfill the wrappers.

Let's begin!

1. Wet the rice paper wrapper under warm running water or dip them in a large bowl of warm water. This softens up the wrapper so you can roll it.

2. Place the rice paper wrapper on a flat smooth surface. Top the wrapper with an assortment of vegetables. Be careful not to overfill. Leave 2 inches free on either side.

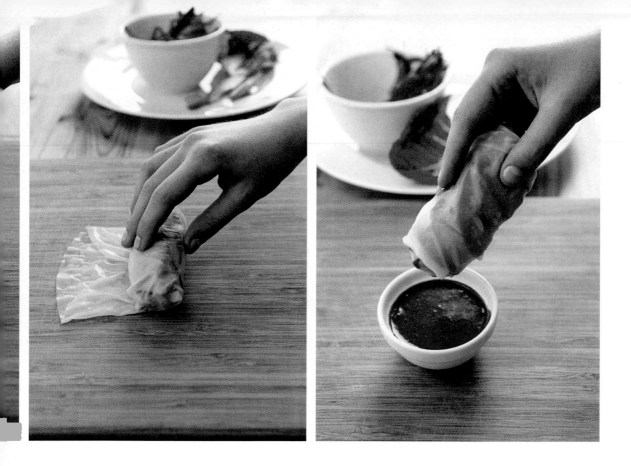

3. Fold up the bottom of the wrapper. The bottom of the wrapper is the part that is closest to you. Fold this up over the filling and press down slightly.

4. Fold in the sides and continue rolling, holding onto the sides as you make the first roll because they are still a little slippery at this point. Once you have the first roll completed, you can let go of the sides and continue rolling the spring roll until you reach the end of the rice paper wrapper.

5. Now dip your spring roll in some Not Peanut Sauce (page 20) and enjoy!

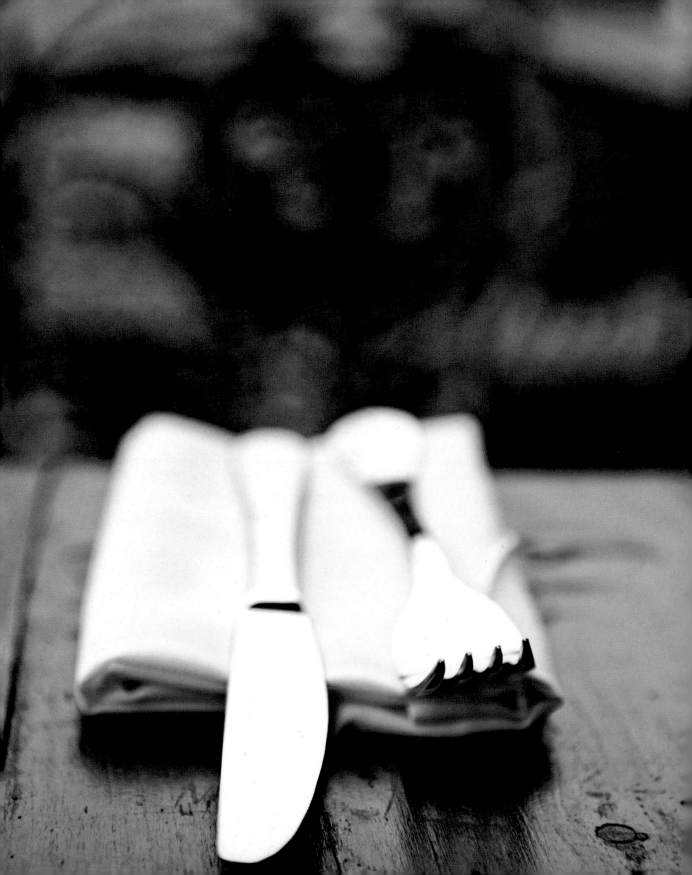

Things Get Heated*

▪ Soothing the Soul ▪

Sunny Slope Farm in Alton, New Hampshire, is a cozy farmhouse retreat where I have created many raw meals for people who come together to refresh their spirits—and in return, refresh my spirit. My first stay at Sunny Slope Farm was a snow-filled week in February—a true winter wonderland. Every day I had a version of this hot creamy soup simmering on the stovetop.

While I promote a diet high in raw foods, a hot cooked soup can do our bodies good. A hot soup will soothe the emotions and provide comfort and sustenance during cold winter months. A diet that is 100% raw is just too rigid for most of us. It's too extreme on our bodies, and can sap our joy. This soup will give you the warming support needed to continue your raw journey.

---

*   *After much debate with my editor about whether or not I could include a cooked food item in a book titled* Eat Raw, Not Cooked, *we still could not come to an agreement. I won the arm-wrestling match (because I drank my Happy Shakes . . .) and am slipping in three recipes that have been crucial to the success my families have had in incorporating a raw food diet into their lives.*

▪ No Vegetable Left Behind ▪

This cooked soup makes great use of parts of vegetables that might otherwise go by the wayside. The perfect example is when making Broccoli Alfredo (page 75), which uses broccoli florets: Save the broccoli stalks for a Creamy Broccoli Cauliflower Soup. When making julienned zucchini noodles (see page 78, step 4), save and throw in the inner seedy parts of the zucchini. Add an onion, carrot, or celery, if you like, for a simply wonderful hot comforting soup!

▪ Sunny Slope Farm Soup ▪

Every time I make this soup it tastes different, depending on what is available. Enjoy being creative by mixing and matching your vegetable and seasoning possibilities. While Sunny Slope Farm Soup has a very rich and buttery flavor, it is also very low in calories, fat, and carbohydrates, making it a dieter's best friend. A cup of soup will run you approximately 50 calories and 7g carbohydrates. Here is a list of basic vegetables—mix and match!

VEGETABLE OPTIONS

zucchini	yams, skin on and sliced	**Seasoning possibilities:**
summer squash	acorn squash, peeled and chopped	organic chicken broth
cauliflower		nutritional yeast flakes
broccoli	butternut squash, peeled and chopped	salt and pepper
carrots		onion or garlic powder
celery	pumpkin, peeled and chopped	cayenne pepper
onion		red pepper flakes

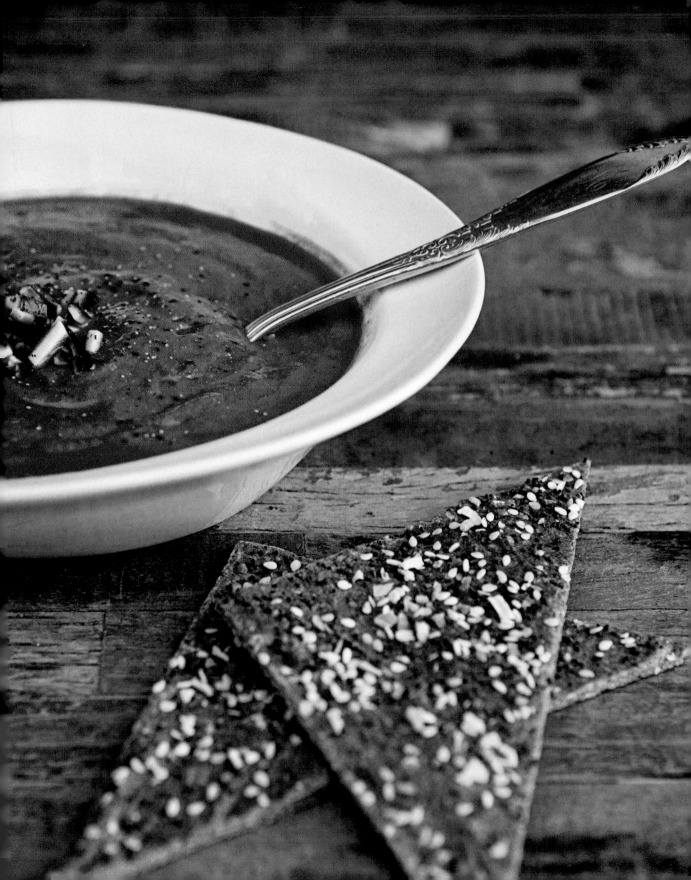

SUNNY SLOPE FARM SOUP

Nutritional yeast flakes will give your soup that buttery rich flavor we love in a cream soup. Add a little more or a little less to suit your taste. It is very important you read the label on your nutritional yeast flakes. This is *not brewer's yeast*. Brewer's yeast will taste horrible. You will end up throwing your pot of soup away, and blaming *me*!

SUGGESTED INGREDIENTS

1 medium head cauliflower
3 medium yellow summer squash
2 celery stalks
2 carrots
½ cup chopped onion
1 cup nutritional yeast flakes
salt and fresh ground pepper, to taste

1. Cut the vegetables for easy boiling. Cover the vegetables in water, cover with a lid, and boil.

2. Once you can pierce the vegetables with a fork, transfer them to a blender with some of the cooking water. Blend until creamy. Transfer back to a pot and add your nutritional yeast flakes, salt, and pepper. You will make your soup thicker or thinner by the amount of cooking water you use.

Note: I have saved much time in blending by using an immersion blender found in most kitchen stores for $30.

SERVINGS: APPROXIMATELY 10

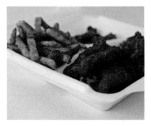

41

LONG JOHN SILVER'S FISH & CHIPS

Fried foods are polluting the average American's diet. Restaurants serve these foods up cheap, fast, and in hefty-size portions. A deep-fried meal of fish and chips can run you 1,000 calories and 55 grams of fat . . . so ditch it! Here are some tips to avoiding these fatty foods:

1. Swap out your favorite fried foods with healthier substitutes. (Trust me, you are going to love my version of fish & chips!)

2. Plan meals ahead of time so there's no last-minute resorting to fast foods—big no-no!

3. Prepare healthy snacks in advance and have them available.

4. Keep a food journal so you can view your progress.

5. Stay away from fast-food chains.

FISH & "CHIPS"

A raw vegan diet works miracles at healing and cleansing, giving many people their lives back, myself included. That said, it's not a diet to live on. There are B12 deficiencies happening within the raw vegan community. This does not mean you can't be a successful raw vegan. You just have to be vigilant with regards to testing your blood and supplementing your diet. My personal choice is to supplement my body with real food. The only sufficient natural food source of vitamin B12 comes from animals, and this is why I have included a pan-seared salmon in these pages.

This recipe makes the tastiest and easiest meal in minutes without smelling up your house like an all-out fish fry. Pan-searing salmon is my very favorite way to prepare fish. Along with this incredibly rich and flaky salmon, I serve raw "chips" made from crisp hearts of romaine. The perfect sauce along side your Fish & "Chips" is the Basic White Sauce (page 22). This sauce has a nice, light lemon-garlic flavor that will not overpower the fish. Add in a little raw pickle relish found in many health food stores, and you have an excellent tartar sauce that is far superior to processed commercial versions. One guilt-free serving of my Fish & "Chips" will run you approximately 250 calories and 9g fat.

2 pieces of salmon fillet (7 ounces each)
Refined coconut oil
Sea salt

1 lemon
Romaine Chips (page 15)
Basic White Sauce (page 22)

1. Remove the skin from the salmon and cut into smaller pieces ¾ inch wide and 3 inches long. These smaller pieces will sear faster and easier, which means less chance of smoking up your kitchen.

2. Heat up a cast iron skillet to medium to high heat on the stovetop. Add a little coconut oil to the hot pan. Lay the salmon pieces in the hot pan and sear until it turns a nice golden brown color and almost cooked through, 3 to 4 minutes depending on how rare or well done you prefer. (Salmon is a nice fish to leave slightly undercooked). Flip the salmon pieces over for a quick 10-second sear on the second side.

3. Sprinkle with a little sea salt. Serve with lemon, romaine chips, and the Basic White Sauce. I enjoy filling romaine chips with salmon, creating little salmon tacos.

SERVES 2

WHAT ARE THE SYMPTOMS OF A VITAMIN B12 DEFICIENCY?

Vitamin B12 is stored in the body for years, so it could take some time before signs of a deficiency show up. However, when it does occur, the symptoms can include low counts of healthy red blood cells, weakness, fatigue, depression, numbness and tingling in the fingers and toes, nerve damage, cognitive changes, loss of appetite, or sore tongue.

What are the best food sources of vitamin B12? This B vitamin is found naturally in animal-based foods such as fish, eggs, poultry, meat, and dairy foods. Two of the richest sources of vitamin B12 are sardines and salmon.

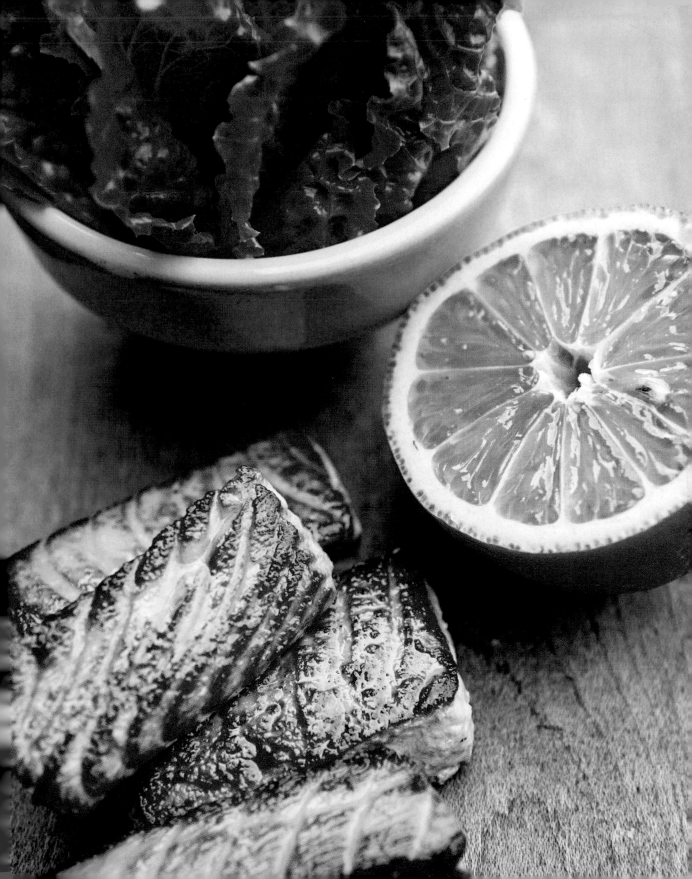

42

LATTE WITH WHIPPED CREAM TOPPING

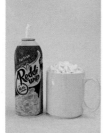

Latte with whipped cream topping—back in the day this was my go-to, after-dinner treat . . . espresso, served with steamed milk and topped with a squirt of "Lite" Cool Whip Topping. Yum!

What exactly is Reddi Wip Topping?

Ingredients: nonfat milk, cream, sugar, corn syrup, inulin (chicory extract), cellulose, mono and diglycerides, polysorbate 80, artificial flavor(s), carrageenan

While there exists some "real cream" as the label states, it also contains a lot of chemicals and air!

See page 135 for my Way Cool Stacy Whip optional topping.

SILVER TEA

Today, I have a new after-dinner go-to. I have brought this treasure into every single one of my family's homes. I would say it is the most important recipe in this whole book. . . .

The amazing power of Silver Tea is that it is something that can be enjoyed socially, yet is almost sacred when savored alone. Silver Tea has a smooth, clean taste, is naturally hydrating, and caffeine-free. Silver Tea is ideal for signaling the end of your meal, and also perfect for starting your morning out right. The best part . . . Silver Tea is *free*!

I have even learned how to order Silver Tea in other countries. For example, in Mexico City, I simply ask, "Agua caliente, por favor?" and out comes a beautiful white teacup and saucer with piping hot water to warm me right up.

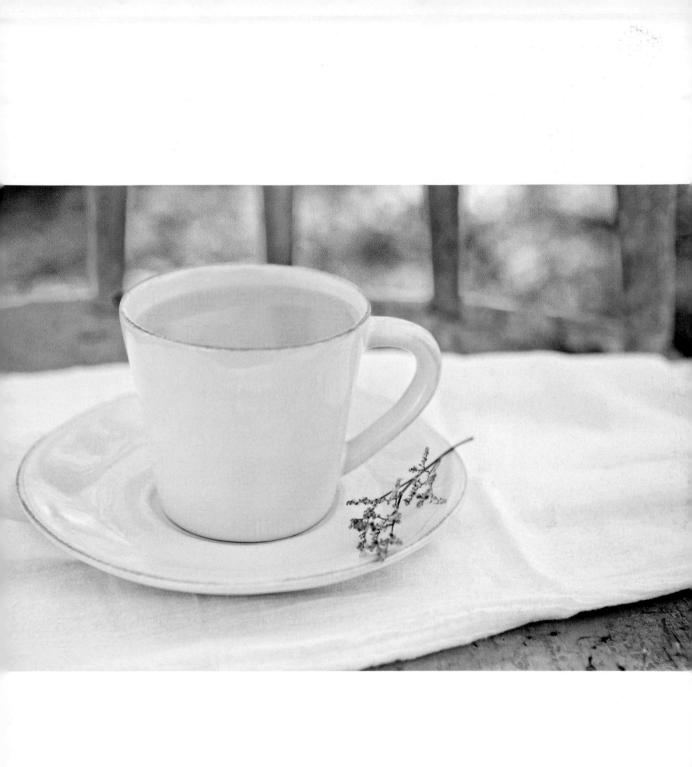

THINGS GET HEATED

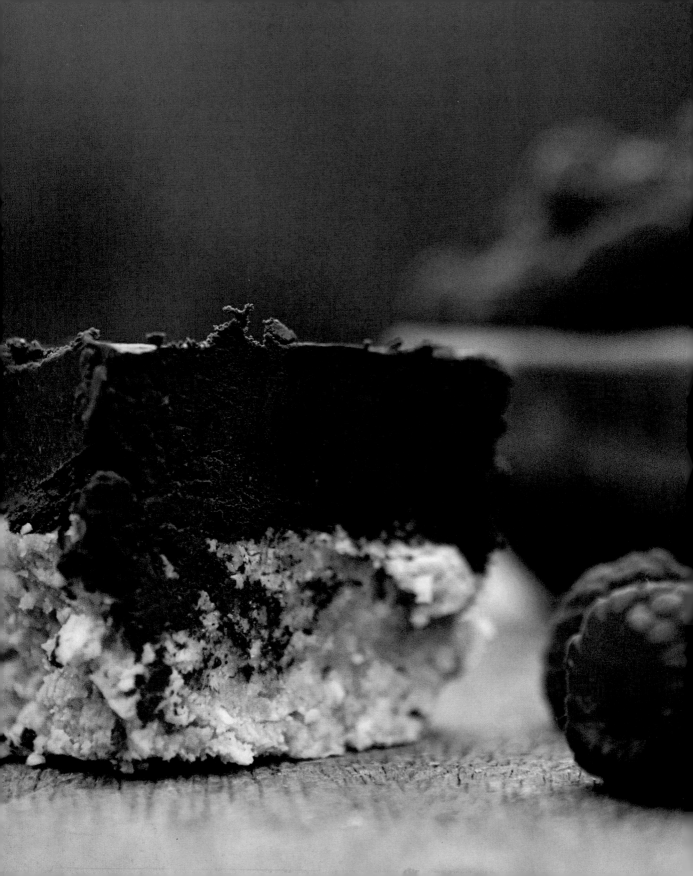

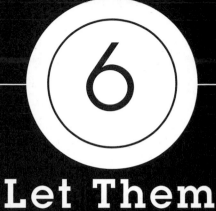

Let Them Eat . . . Dessert!

PIES

Coconut Banana Cream Pie

Chunky Monkey Pie

Chocolate Pecan Pie

Kimmie's Key Lime Pie

"Almond Joy" Pie

Blueberry Land Cheesecake

Cinderella Pumpkin Pie

Peace Out Chocolate Cake

Jacob's Summer Peach Cobbler

MOUSSE & PUDDING

Vermont Joe's Chocolate Moose

Cha-Cha-Chia Pudding

SAUCES & SYRUPS

Wicked Caramel Sauce

Chocolate Ganache

ICE CREAM TREAT

Banana Road Kill

MILK & COOKIES

Just Almond Milk

Stacy Doodles

Mini Me's

Sarah Bernhardt Cookie, Gone Raw!

Hard Chocolate . . . for Chocolate-Covered Everything!

Cioffi Bars

Chocolate Macaroon Fudge Bars

"Peanut Butter" Freezer Cookies

Chocolate Donut Holes

Truffles for Sue

Chocolate Chip Cookie Dough Balls

Jimmy Chews

Y ou are going to *love* this chapter! You get to eat dessert with no guilt. First of all, you haven't filled yourself up with a heavy starchy dinner. You feel light and energized, the way our fuel, or our food, should leave us feeling. Second, these desserts are all made with ingredients that are not simply for amusing our mouths: They are good for us. The beauty of making desserts with ingredients that are highly dense in nutrition is that you will not be drawn to overconsume. Food that is nutritious satisfies. I have worked with many people who lost weight enjoying raw desserts. This is why my families will often hear me quip: "Let them eat pie!"

THE SCOOP ON SUGAR

There is a difference between consuming naturally occurring plant sugars (fructose) and the sugar (sucrose) found in granulated white sugar and high fructose corn syrup often used to sweeten processed foods. Granulated sugar and high fructose corn syrup go through a refining process. These sugars are considered "empty calories," providing no nutritional benefits. These processed sugars are highly addictive and rob your body of health and vitality. Whole foods that contain naturally occurring sugars, like dates, raw honey, and fruit are going to be higher in nutritional value than what's found (or more accurately, what's not found) in all the empty calories we eat from the processed foods.

TRADITIONAL COOKED BANANA CREAM PIE

A cooked banana cream pie can taste fantastic, but is full of saturated fat, whole milk, shortening, and trans fat. These are the fats we don't want. When it comes to fat, trans fat is considered to be the worst type of fat. Trans fat occurs when oils are processed into solid fats. Trans fat both raises your "bad" (LDL) cholesterol and lowers your "good" (HDL) cholesterol. A high-LDL cholesterol level in combination with a low-HDL cholesterol level increases your risk of heart disease, the leading killer of men and women. Here are just some of the products that many times contain trans fats:

- Cookies
- Crackers
- Cakes
- Muffins
- Pie crusts
- Pizza dough

- Margarine
- Vegetable shortening
- Cake mixes
- Pancake mixes
- Chocolate drink mixes
- Donuts

- French fries
- Potato chips
- Candy
- Packaged popcorn
- Frozen dinners

COCONUT BANANA CREAM PIE

This all-time favorite pie was first devoured by the Wells family. I had never had coconut cream pie before I met them, and since it was Rod's favorite dessert, I asked him to describe it to me. After much discussion over the fact that this pie could easily be thrown in someone's face should the need arise, I created Coconut Banana Cream Pie—thank you for the inspiration, Rod. You have made many a family very happy!

CRUST
1 cup raw almonds
1 cup finely shredded coconut
1 cup packed pitted Medjool dates (10 to 12)
⅛ teaspoon salt
1 tablespoon water, if needed

FILLING
1½ cups canned organic coconut milk (see Note)
2 ripe bananas, cut into chunks

½ cup pitted Medjool dates (5 to 6)
Pinch of salt
1 teaspoon pure vanilla extract
1 tablespoon lecithin
½ cup unrefined coconut oil

GARNISH
1 banana, thinly sliced
2 tablespoons finely shredded coconut

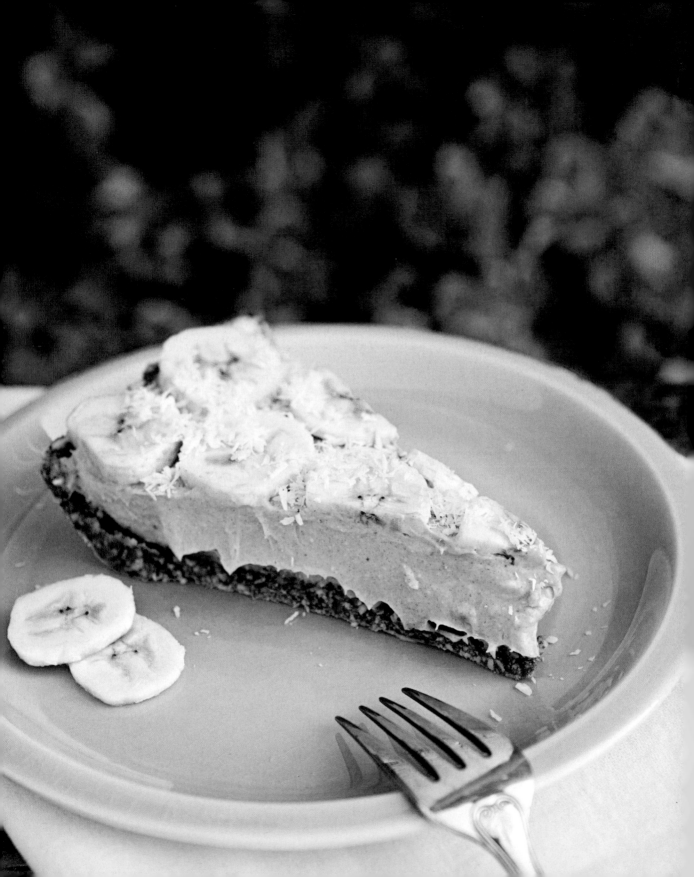

1. For the crust: In a blender, combine all the ingredients and process until the ingredients stick together. Don't overprocess or you will make nut butter. Press the mixture into a pie plate. Chill while preparing your pie filling.

2. For the filling: In a blender, combine the coconut milk, bananas, dates, salt, and vanilla and blend well. Add the lecithin and coconut oil and blend again. Pour the filling over your pie crust. Chill for 8 hours.

3. Decorate with the bananas and some sprinkles of shredded coconut.

SERVES 8

Note: This amount is a bit less than the whole can. Never use "lite" coconut milk.

Little Brother Richie's Banana Tip: Use frozen bananas in the filling mixture for faster chilling.

COCONUT OIL

Coconut oil is beneficial for the heart. It is about 50% lauric acid, which helps in preventing high blood pressure and high cholesterol. Coconut oil does not lead to an increase in "bad" (LDL) cholesterol levels and actually aids in weight loss. Most people notice that after adding coconut oil into their diets, they are less prone to snacking.

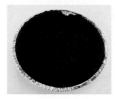

44

KEEBLER® CHOCOLATE READY CRUST

Let's take a look at the crust. . . .

Ingredients: Enriched Flour (Wheat Flour, Niacin, Reduced Iron, Thiamin Mononitrate, Riboflavin, Folic Acid), **Sugar**, Partially Hydrogenated Soybean Oil, Cocoa, **Corn Syrup**, contains 2% or less of Molasses, Salt, Chocolate, Leavening (Baking Soda, Sodium Acid Pyrophosphate, Monocalcium Phospate), Malt, Cornstarch, Soy Lecithin.

~⁀⁀

CHUNKY MONKEY PIE

. . . . with the best chocolate walnut brownie crust ever!

This pie came about with my Long Island, New York family. Marisol wanted a chocolate dessert and David wanted a banana dessert. So I went to work combining the two, gave my new creation a cute name, and Chunky Monkey Pie became an instant hit! The crust is a moist rich chocolate walnut brownie. I top this pie with strawberries, shredded coconut, and Chocolate Ganache (page 150), which turns it into a true delight for the eyes as well as the mouth!

CRUST
1½ cups packed pitted Medjool dates
1 cup raw cacao powder
1 cup raw almonds
½ cup raw cashews
⅛ teaspoon salt
1 tablespoon pure vanilla extract
7 tablespoons water
½ cup chopped walnuts

FILLING
1 cup canned organic coconut milk
1 cup raw cashews (see Note)

½ cup raw honey
1 tablespoon pure vanilla extract
1 tablespoon fresh lemon juice
Pinch of salt
2 tablespoons lecithin
½ cup unrefined coconut oil
2 bananas, 1 cut into chunks, 1 sliced

TOPPING
1 cup strawberry chunks
1 banana, cut into chunks
¼ cup shredded coconut
Chocolate Ganache (page 150), optional

1. For the crust: In a food processor, combine the dates, cacao powder, almonds, cashews, salt, vanilla, water, and walnuts and process until you get a thick, moist brownie that holds together. (You may need to add additional water or dates. Buying the juiciest dates possible is helpful.) Press the mixture into a pie plate and chill while preparing the pie filling.

2. For the filling: In a blender, combine the coconut milk, cashews, honey, vanilla, lemon juice, and salt and blend. Add in the lecithin and coconut oil and blend again. Stir in the banana chunks.

3. Layer the pie crust with the sliced banana and pour the filling over the banana-topped pie crust. Chill for 8 hours.

4. Decorate with the strawberries, bananas, and Chocolate Ganache, if using. Top with some sprinkles of shredded coconut and—voilà, Chunky Monkey Pie!

SERVES 8

Note: If you don't have a high-powered blender like a Vitamix, soak the cashews for at least 2 hours or overnight in the refrigerator. Rinse in clean water.

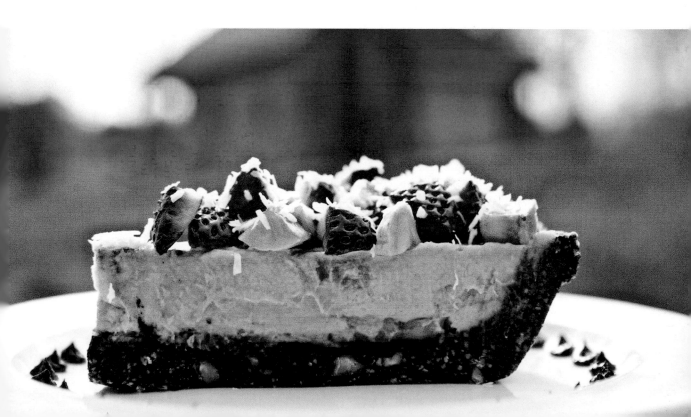

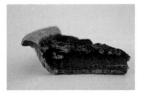

45

HOMEMADE SOUTHERN PECAN PIE

What's in a pecan pie? Unsalted butter, vegetable shortening, all-purpose flour, sugar, eggs, dark corn syrup, vanilla extract, pecans.

It's easy to binge on high-fat, high-sugar, "empty-calorie" baked desserts. This is because endorphins are released that give us those happy feelings when we eat these things. Ever have that intense craving for a plate of slice-and-bake chocolate chip cookies after an argument with your boyfriend? Or that sigh of relief when you bite into a hot fudge sundae? Endorphins.

Studies have shown that there are three dietary triggers that directly lead to the release of endorphins: fats, sugars, and phenylethylamine (PEA). The beauty of raw desserts is that the fats and sugar come in nutrient-rich ingredients, making them extremely satisfying and difficult to binge on. As far as PEA goes, it comes from eating raw chocolate, so you can have this happy feeling every morning in your Happy Shake (page 3)!

"DATE" FACTS

One Medjool date is equal to 167mg of potassium. Potassium is helpful in controlling heart rate and blood pressure, so dates offer protection against stroke and coronary heart disease.

Just one date has 66 calories and 18g carbohydrates. Given that dates contain a large amount of micronutrients and beneficial compounds, these calories are not "empty calories" that are found in most pies, cakes, and cookies.

During the Ramadan holy month in Arab countries, dates are commonly consumed after breaking fast. They replenish energy and revitalize the body instantly, as the natural sugars, sucrose, glucose, and fructose provide tons of energy perfect for breaking a fast, or taking a run. The calcium and magnesium in dates ensures healthy bones and teeth.

Avoid laxatives, eat dates! Medjool dates are an excellent source of fiber. Just two dates have 3.2g of fiber in them. This is the perfect serving if you are trying to increase your fiber intake.

CHOCOLATE PECAN PIE

. . . in honor of the Martha's Vineyard Annual Fishing Derby!

Have you ever heard of Derby Pie? Derby Pie is a pastry that was created at the Melrose Inn in Prospect, Kentucky, by the Kern family and is associated with the Kentucky Derby. The recipe is a highly guarded secret and I have only heard stories about this amazing pie, so I did my best to re-create this chocolaty pecan treat. So when my family on the Vineyard were gearing up for the Martha's Vineyard Annual Fishing Derby, I decided to re-create this chocolate, pecan, caramel delight . . . and boy did I! The best compliment came from my 14-year-old dinner guest, Gordon, who without looking up from his pie said, "Mom, you gotta get this recipe." You got it, Gordon, my pleasure!

CRUST

¾ cup raw almonds

1 cup raw pecans

1 cup packed pitted Medjool dates (10 to 12)

⅛ teaspoon salt

¼ teaspoon ground cinnamon

1 tablespoon water, if needed

GANACHE & FILLING

Chocolate Ganache (page 150)

1⅓ cups canned organic coconut milk

½ cup raw pecans (see Note)

1 cup pitted Medjool dates

⅛ teaspoon salt

1 tablespoon lecithin

Pecans, for garnish

1. For the crust: In a food processor, process all the ingredients until they stick together. Don't overprocess or you will make nut butter. Press the mixture into a pie plate. Chill while you make the ganache.

2. Spread the crust with ½ cup of the Chocolate Ganache, covering the bottom and the sides. This way you get chocolate in every bite! (The ganache recipe makes more than you need. Save the remaining ganache for decorating if you like. You will need to thin it out with a little water for drizzling.)

3. For the filling: In a blender, combine the coconut milk, pecans, dates, and salt and blend until smooth and creamy. Add the lecithin and continue to blend. Pour the filling into the chocolate-covered crust and chill for 4 to 6 hours.

4. Decorate with pecans and Chocolate Ganache once chilled and firm.

Note: Soak the raw pecans for the filling for 4 hours and rinse thoroughly. This will make blending them into creamy goodness a breeze, while releasing those pesky little enzyme inhibitors, making it easier for your body to digest. If you are in a state of pie emergency and are using a high-speed, 2.5-horsepower blender, no worries on soaking your nuts.

SERVES 8

THE RAW NUT

Most of us love nuts! They are tasty, handy, satisfying, and sustaining. We feel great eating them because they are so good for us, notable for being high in omega-3 fats.

Don't roast your nuts! The problem with roasting nuts is that their healthy oils are vulnerable to light, heat, and oxidation. Once you heat the healthy oils found in nuts, you degrade them. The plus side for the manufacturers is that roasting nuts gives these oils a longer shelf life. Expect more from your nuts: eat raw, not cooked.

And for a simple, delicious treat, try this recipe for Salted Caramel Pecan Crunch: Pinch open a sweet juicy Medjool date. Remove the pit and replace it with a raw pecan. Sprinkle with salt. Enjoy anytime for a quick salted caramel pecan fix!

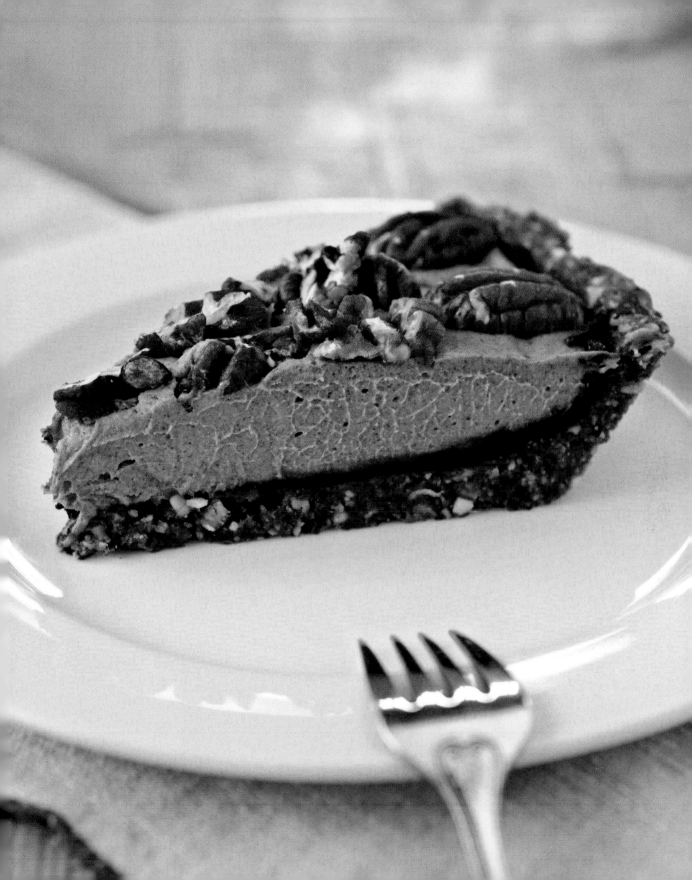

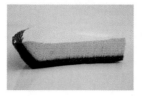

EDWARDS® KEY LIME PIE

Can you pronounce what's in a slice of Edwards Key Lime Pie?

Ingredients: Milk Condensed Reduced Fat Sweetened (Milk, Milk Skim, Sugar, Vitamin A Palmitate), Water, Vegetable(s) Shortening Partially Hydrogenated (Palm Kernel Oil, Soybean(s) Oil, Coconut Oil), Flour Enriched (Wheat Flour, Niacin, Iron Reduced, Thiamine Mononitrate (Vitamin B1), Riboflavin (Vitamin B2), Folic Acid (Vitamin B9)), Sugar, High Fructose Corn Syrup, Egg(s) Yolks, contains 2% or less of the following: Food Starch Modified, Lime Pulp, Baking Soda, Lime Oil, Lime Juice Concentrate, Bleached Enriched Flour (Wheat Flour Bleached, Barley Malted Flour, Niacin, Iron Reduced, Thiamine Mononitrate (Vitamin B1), Riboflavin (Vitamin B2), Folic Acid (Vitamin B9)), Salt, Flavor(s) Natural & Artificial, Dextrose, Lemon(s) Juice Concentrate, Sodium Citrate, Sodium Caseinate, Methylcellulose Hydroxypropyl, Polysorbate 60, Soy Lecithin, Beta Carotene, Xanthan Gum, Disodium Phosphate, Polyglycerol Esters Of Fatty Acids, Lemon(s) Pulp Cells, Guar Gum, Lemon(s) Oil, Sorbitan Monostearate.

'Nuf said!

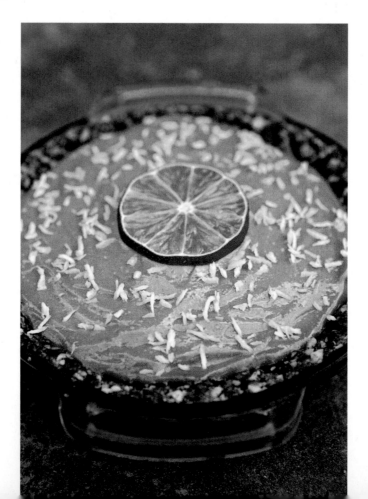

KIMMIE'S KEY LIME PIE

This pie is an all-time family favorite and it only takes minutes to make. You will be shocked by the simplicity of the ingredients: limes and avocado. The avocado is what gives this lime pie its beautiful green color and wonderful creamy consistency. I promise: You will never taste the avocado. Avocados are bursting with nutrients: vitamins A, B vitamins (including folate and biotin), C, E, and K; plus minerals such as magnesium, copper, iron, calcium, and potassium. They provide all 18 essential aminos, making this fruit a complete protein. Avocados are also rich in seven fatty acids, including omega-3 and omega-6, and are a complete protein, easy to digest and readily absorbed by the body. The avocado is extremely rich and satisfying, so if you are trying to move to a more vegetable-based diet, it can be your new best ally.

CRUST
¾ cup raw almonds
1 cup raw walnuts
1 cup packed pitted Medjool dates (10 to 12)
⅛ teaspoon salt
1 tablespoon water, if needed

FILLING
¾ cup fresh lime juice
1½ cups avocados
½ cup raw honey
½ teaspoon pure vanilla extract
⅛ teaspoon salt
2 tablespoons lecithin
½ cup unrefined coconut oil
Fresh berries, kiwi or lime slices, and shredded coconut, for garnish, optional

1. **For the crust:** In a food processor, process all the ingredients until they stick together. Don't overprocess or you will make nut butter. Press the crust mixture into a pie plate. Chill while preparing the pie filling.

2. **For the filling:** In a blender, combine the lime juice, avocados, honey, vanilla, and salt and blend well. Add the lecithin and coconut oil and blend again until creamy. Pour the filling into the crust. Chill for 6 to 8 hours or until firm.

3. Garnish with a slice of lime or kiwi fruit or colorful berries, and shredded coconut, if using.

SERVES 8

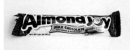

47

HOMEMADE ALMOND JOY PIE

Here are the ingredients for a homemade pie made with Almond Joy candy bars (based on a recipe found on a website): A LOT of Almond Joy bars (36 miniatures), graham crackers, sugar, cornstarch, cocoa powder, salt, milk, vanilla.

What is in an Almond Joy Miniature? Corn Syrup, Milk Chocolate (Sugar, Cocoa Butter, Chocolate, Milk, Lactose, Milkfat, Nonfat Milk, and Soy Lecithin and PGPR, Emulsifiers), Coconut, Sugar, Almonds; contains 2% or less of: Partially Hydrogenated Vegetable Oil (Cottonseed and Soybean Oil), Whey (Milk), Cocoa, Salt, Natural and Artificial Flavor, Chocolate, Hydrolyzed Milk Protein, Soy Lecithin, Carmel Color, Sodium Metabisulfite, and Sulfur Dioxide.

This doesn't sound so "homemade," does it?

"ALMOND JOY" PIE

"Sometimes you feel like a nut, sometimes you don't." I grew up with this jingle. Personally, I always felt like a nut! In this pie, I have recaptured this old familiar comfort food. I hope it takes you back.

CRUST	FILLING
1 cup raw almonds	1 can (13.5 ounces) organic coconut milk
1 cup finely shredded coconut	3 tablespoons raw cacao
1 cup packed pitted Medjool dates (10 to 12)	¾ cup cashews (see Note)
⅛ teaspoon salt	1 cup plus 3 Medjool dates
1 tablespoon water, if needed	⅛ teaspoon salt
	2 tablespoons lecithin

GARNISH:
Raw almonds and shredded coconut

1. For the crust: In a food processor, process all the ingredients until they stick together. Don't overprocess or you will make nut butter. Press the crust mixture into a pie plate. Chill while preparing the pie filling.

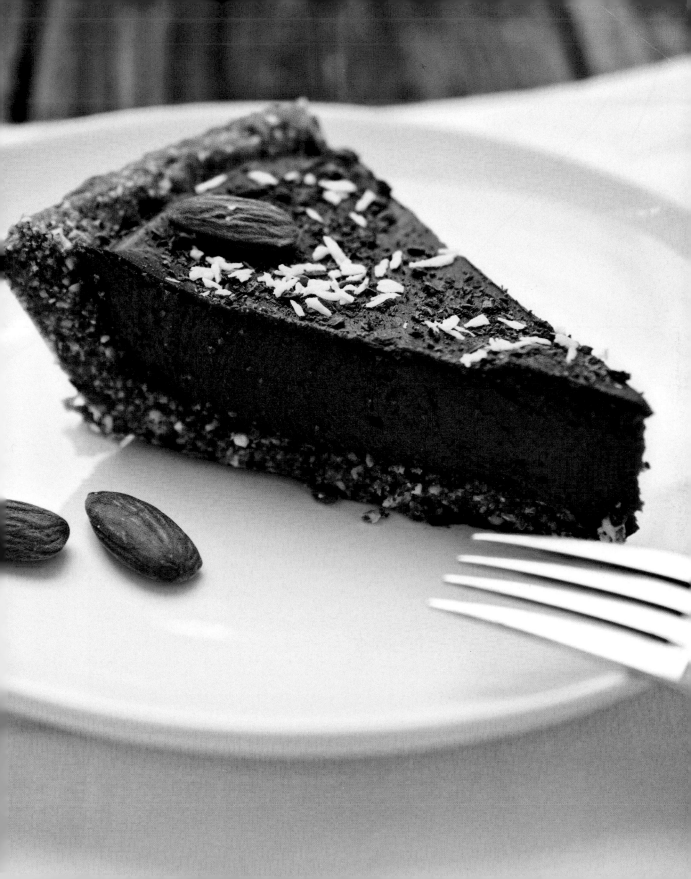

2. For the filling: In a blender, combine the coconut milk, cacao, cashews, dates, and salt and blend until creamy. Add the lecithin and blend again. Pour the filling into the crust. Chill for 6 to 8 hours.

3. Decorate with the shredded coconut and almonds.

SERVES 8

Note: Unless you're using a high-speed blender such as a Vitamix, soak the cashews for at least 2 hours before blending. Rinse them thoroughly after soaking.

ALMONDS, CHOCOLATE, AND COCONUT!

Here are just three reasons I love this combination:

1. Raw almonds help reduce the rise in blood sugar and insulin levels after meals. This offers protection against diabetes. Raw almonds also have tons of fiber, helping to prevent constipation. Be sure to drink plenty of water when eating this much fiber.

2. Stressed? Raw cacao contains significant amounts of tryptophan. This nutrient is a mood-elevating powerhouse. Tryptophan in turn produces serotonin. Serotonin builds our "stress-defense shield." Nothing can bring us down if serotonin levels are high. Note that tryptophan is heat sensitive, so a processed chocolate bar just isn't going to cut it. You must eat your chocolate raw, not cooked, in order to get this happy tool.

3. Dairy products are made up of long-chain saturated fats. These fats are cholesterol-heavy and high in calories. Coconut milk, by contrast, is made up of saturated fats containing mostly medium-chain fatty acids, which the body can metabolize efficiently and convert pretty quickly into energy.

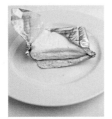

CHEESECAKE

Cheesecake is one of the worst foods for anyone trying to avoid a heart attack—which is all of us! Loaded with full-fat cream cheese, butter, heavy whipping cream, sour cream, and egg yolks, cheesecake, along with the rest of your high-fat diet, can eventually kill you.

Heart disease is the #1 killer of Americans every year. Why? Because we are eating ourselves to death. Heart disease can be prevented and cured by simply changing our diets. Not so simple—this means giving up our food addictions.

BLUEBERRY LAND CHEESECAKE

Blueberries, blueberries, blueberries—all I see are blueberries! This was what I was thinking as I met the Whitney Family in Machias, Maine. They have been growing and supplying blueberries for four generations, and I happened to be in Blueberry Land at the peak of blueberry picking season—I was in luck! Because most families own pie plates, this recipe is designed to create a quick and simple pie version of a cheesecake instead of calling for a springform pan.

CRUST
¾ cup raw almonds
1 cup raw walnuts
1 cup packed pitted Medjool dates (10 to 12)
⅛ teaspoon salt
1 tablespoon water, if needed

FILLING
1 cup raw cashews (see Note)
½ cup raw honey

½ cup fresh lemon juice
4 pitted Medjool dates (¼ cup)
1½ tablespoons lecithin
½ cup unrefined coconut oil

BLUEBERRY SAUCE
3 cups blueberries
1 tablespoon raw honey
1 tablespoon fresh lemon juice

1. For the crust: In a food processor, process all the ingredients until they stick together. Don't overprocess or you will make nut butter. Press the crust mixture into a pie plate. Chill while preparing the pie filling.

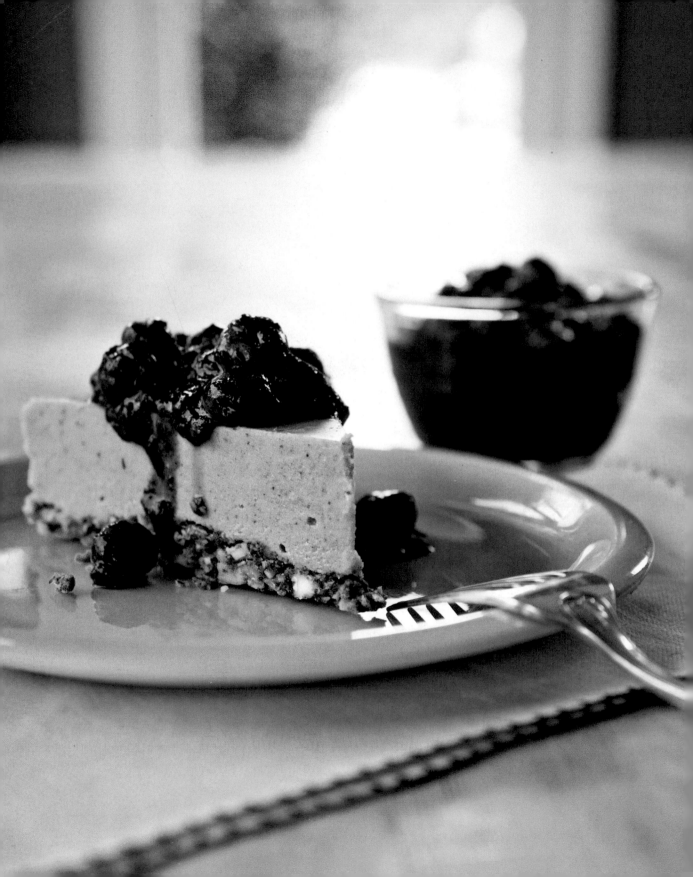

2. For the filling: In a blender, combine the cashews, honey, lemon juice, and dates and blend. Add the lecithin and coconut oil and blend again. Pour the filling into the crust. Chill for 6 to 8 hours.

3. For the sauce: In a blender, combine 1 cup of the blueberries, the honey, and lemon juice and blend. Pour into a bowl and stir in the remaining 2 cups blueberries.

4. Serve the cheesecake topped with the blueberry sauce.

SERVES 8

Note: Unless you're using a high-speed blender such as a Vitamix, soak the cashews for at least 2 hours before blending. Rinse them thoroughly after soaking.

BLUEBERRIES

North America supplies up to 90% of the world's blueberries. Plump full of antioxidants (those free-radical-fighting powerhouses that help prevent damage to your body's cells), blueberries have been ranked the #1 fruit for antioxidants. They are low in calories, too—fewer than 100 calories per cup. (For a true blueberry experience, head up to Machias, Maine, where the blueberry is celebrated throughout July at the peak of its harvest, during National Blueberry Month.)

THE HEART-HEALTHY CASHEW

The fat in cashews comes in the form of oleic acid, the same heart-healthy monounsaturated fat found in olive oil. Studies have shown that oleic acid promotes a healthy cardiovascular system by reducing triglyceride levels. Cashews are loaded with antioxidants, preventing heart disease. The magnesium found in cashews helps lower blood pressure and ward off heart attacks. Coconut oil is a staple in many native Pacific tropical islands. Studies have shown these people have a nearly nonexistent rate of heart disease.

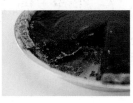

49

BAKERS SQUARE PUMPKIN PIE

While the Bakers Square Pumpkin Pie recipe seems to be top secret, I guarantee, you will never get the same fresh taste of pumpkin from a cooked pie, like you do in my raw version.

CINDERELLA PUMPKIN PIE

Walking through a farmers' market, I stumbled across the most beautiful pumpkin. It was the Cinderella Pumpkin—it looked just like the pumpkin that Cinderella's fairy godmother transformed into a carriage. This pumpkin is perfect for pie—and also goes great in the creamy Sunny Slope Farm Soup (page 108). If you cannot find this particular pumpkin, no worries, any little pumpkin will do.

CRUST	**FILLING**
¾ cup raw almonds	2 cups raw cubed pumpkin
1 cup raw pecans	⅓ cup Grade B maple syrup
1 cup packed pitted Medjool dates (10 to 12)	1 teaspoon fresh lemon juice
⅛ teaspoon salt	1½ teaspoons pumpkin pie spice
1 tablespoon water, if needed	Pinch of sea salt
	⅓ cup unrefined coconut oil
	1 tablespoon lecithin
	Pumpkin seeds, for garnish

1. For the crust: In a food processor, process all the ingredients until they stick together. Don't overprocess or you will make nut butter. Press the crust mixture into a pie plate. Chill while preparing the pie filling.

2. For the filling: In a high-speed blender or food processor, combine the pumpkin, maple syrup, lemon juice, pumpkin pie spice, and sea salt, and process until smooth and creamy. Add the coconut oil and lecithin and blend or process. Pour the filling into the crust. Chill for 6 to 8 hours. Garnish the top with pumpkin seeds.

SERVES 8

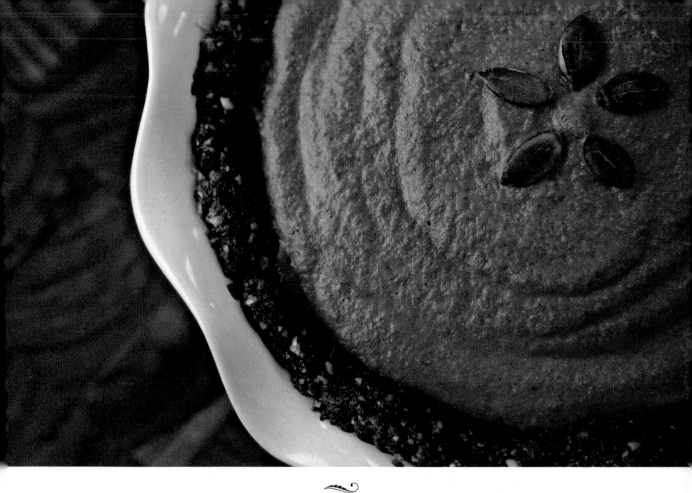

TOPPING OPTION: WAY COOL STACY WHIP

2010: Darren and Bronwin Rhodes were my very first family to open their doors to me, welcoming me in to feed them. That week was my most challenging week ever. It was my first week on the job! By the end of the week we had all fallen in love, and nothing to me is better than the love of family. That was when I knew feeding families was the job best suited for me.

Four years later, I have returned to feed Darren and Bronwin, and now their little yoga baby, Dagda. With a new family member to win over, I have all-new happy baby creations to invent. So as I work in my family's Tucson home, I am both creating new flavors and editing my manuscript for *Eat Raw, Not Cooked* with a deadline in sight! I must share with you the last recipe to be included in the book, the icing on the cake . . . or better yet, the Stacy Whip on the pie!!!

This recipe is dedicated to you Darren, Bronwin, and Dagda. Thank you.

2 cans of Native Valley Organic Coconut Milk (never the "lite" version)

¼ cup raw honey

1 tablespoon vanilla

Pinch of fine sea salt

1 tablespoon lecitin

1. Chill 2 cans of coconut milk in the refrigerator for 8 hours, with the cans standing upright so the thick, white milk solids will reach the top of the cans. There will be a gray, watery liquid on the bottom of the thick white milk. This thin, watery liquid will not give you the consistency of a whip topping. Throw this part away or use it in a future smoothie.

2. In your blender, spoon in the thick, white coconut milk solids from your cans, leaving the gray, watery liquid behind. Add all other ingredients. Blend on high for about 5 seconds.

3. Chill for 12 hours in the refrigerator and allow whip to thicken. Your Way Cool Stacy Whip will be ready for the pie the next day.

SAVE THE PUMPKINS!

Pumpkins are not just for carving up and posting on your doorstep every fall. Their bright color is a dead giveaway that they are chock full of goodness! Being a superfood, the raw pumpkin is full of vitamins A, C, K, and E, and loaded with antioxidant carotenoids, plus loads of minerals, including magnesium, potassium, and iron.

Funnily enough, right when cold and flu season hits, the pumpkin pops up to save the day! Full of beta-carotene, pumpkin reinforces your immune system and protects against colds, flu, and infections. Pumpkins stored in a cool dry place can last up to six months. So load up on this amazing superfood for maximum benefits.

50

STORE-BOUGHT CHOCOLATE BROWNIE

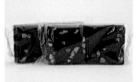

The manufacturing of chocolate means heating the cacao beans to approximately 250°F, a process that destroys the world's most powerful superfood, known for centuries as "the food of the Gods." This means you should not expect to get all the perks you get when eating raw chocolate. Processed chocolate is often paired with refined sugars and fats that may initially give you a high, but which will be followed quickly by a low. This results in reaching for more, eating more, and putting on more weight. Next time you find yourself reaching for chocolate, eat raw, not cooked!

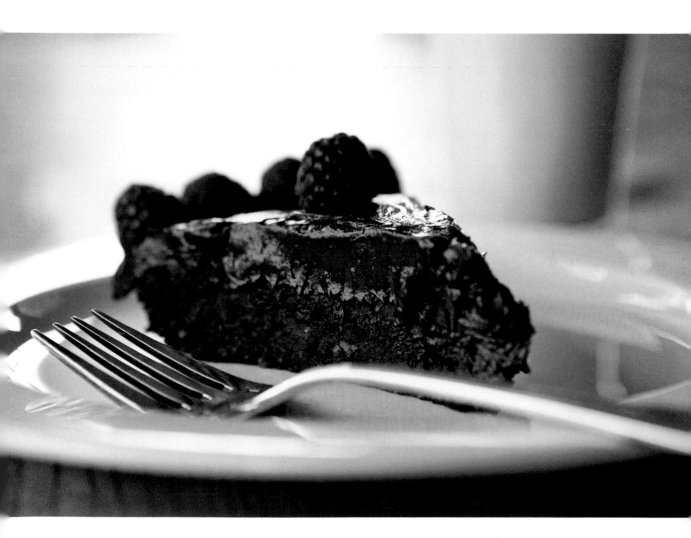

LET THEM EAT . . . DESSERT!

PEACE OUT CHOCOLATE CAKE

Something about food, and especially whole, rich, nourishing foods shared together, bonds people. My favorite way to end the week is with Peace Out Chocolate Cake—you are going to love this very rich brownielike cake. I call it "cake" because "Peace Out Chocolate Brownie" just doesn't sound as cool.

1½ cups raw walnuts

1 cup packed pitted Medjool dates (10 to 12)

⅓ cup raw cacao powder

1 teaspoon pure vanilla extract

⅛ teaspoon salt

1 tablespoon water, if needed

Vermont Joe's Chocolate Moose (page 144)

Garnish: raspberries

1. In a food processor, combine the walnuts, dates, cacao powder, vanilla, and salt. Process until the ingredients stick together. Don't overprocess or you will make nut butter. Press the crust mixture into a pie plate.

2. Top the crust with Vermont Joe's Chocolate Moose and decorate with raspberries in the shape of a peace sign. Peace Out!

SERVES 8

WHY DO I LOVE RAW CHOCOLATE SO MUCH?

Chocolate is all LOVE. Grumpy people don't eat chocolate. Chemically, raw chocolate really is the world's perfect food. There is a very powerful class of compounds found in abundance in raw cacao (pronounced "kuh-KOW") that are not found in cooked chocolate. These compounds are PEAs (short for phenylethylamines). PEAs are a major class of chemicals that we produce in our bodies when we fall in love. PEAs do some other pretty amazing things as well—they increase focus and alertness, while serving as a natural appetite suppressant.

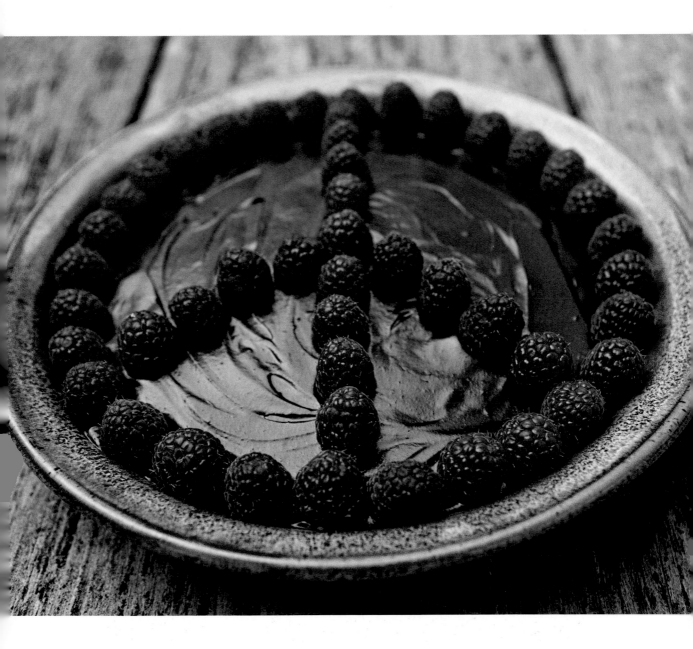

LET THEM EAT . . . DESSERT!

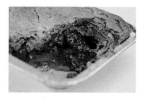

51

MARIE CALLENDER'S® PEACH COBBLER

Modified starches are used for everything from forming jellybean shells to replacing fat in low-fat salami to thickening wallpaper glue. They serve as thickening agents. The big question: Are they bad for you?

Research does not indicate that modified starches are bad for you. They are, however, starches and will increase your blood sugar levels, resulting in weight gain. Note that many foods containing these starches tend to be highly processed foods loaded in sodium, fat, and sugar— "empty calories." The goal? Make every calorie count!

Filling Ingredients: Peaches, Sugar, Water, **Modified Food Starch**, Salt, Ascorbic Acid And Citric Acid (to Promote Color Retention).

Crust Ingredients: Enriched Wheat Flour (Flour, Niacin, Iron, Thiamin Mononitrate, Riboflavin, Folic Acid), Vegetable Shortening (Partially Hydrogenated Soybean Oil), Water, Dextrose, Salt. Contains Wheat, Soybean.

MEET JACOB

Jacob's parents would say Jacob is the most wonderful kid in the world . . . a beautiful, intelligent, happy, playful, sensitive, active, and loving boy, who is nonverbal due to his autism. Though they communicate through the heart, Jacob's parents have never yet had a conversation with Jacob, to ask what he'd like to eat, or what he did today, or if he's not feeling well. As Jacob's parents, Derrill and Jo-Ann would love to have a simple conversation like that with Jacob, to hear what he's thinking and know what he's feeling. Like any parents, Derrill and Jo-Ann want to see him reach his full potential. No more and no less.

During my week with my new family, I watched as they used a program with Jacob called The Son-Rise Program. Instead of bringing Jacob into their world, they joined Jacob in his activities. The idea is that as a connection with Jacob is made, he would want to join his family in "their world." Jacob lives in a world of balls and he is quite talented with them.

Jacob was an easy boy for me to feed. Everything I brought to him made him happy. Although I enjoyed feeding Jacob, I never really felt a connection. But on my last morning, I went to Jacob's playroom without treats, simply to say goodbye, and this smart little boy knew I was leaving and started bringing me balls. Big balls, little balls, red balls, yellow balls—Jacob was inviting me into his world. I had connected with him through the gift of food! And I promised him I would be back in "70 sleeps"—a promise I was excited to keep.

To learn more about The Son-Rise Program go to www.autismtreatmentcenter.org.

JACOB'S SUMMER PEACH COBBLER

When I first walk into my families' kitchens, my eyes automatically search out any fresh fruits, vegetables, or herbs. I also love to find out what is growing in the garden. The first thing I noticed in Derrill and Jo-Ann's home was a huge bowl of summer-fresh peaches on the kitchen counter. It turns out they came from their ten-year-old son Jacob's very own backyard peach tree, which was planted in honor of his birth. The fruit tasted like heaven! Growing up in the South, my thoughts turned to my great grandmother's Summer Peach Cobbler . . . .

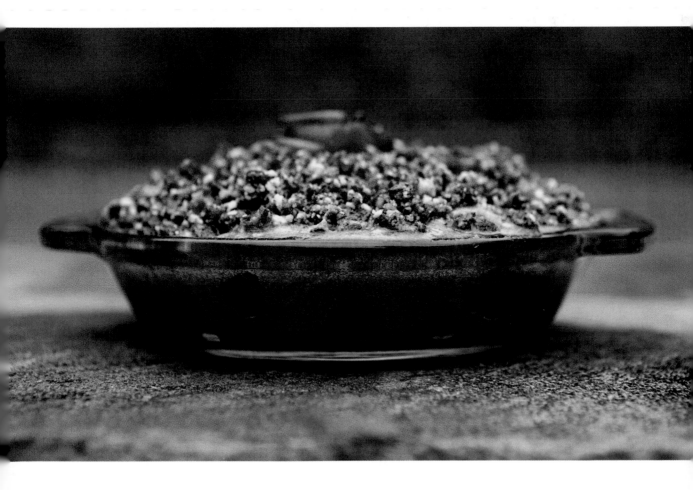

FILLING	TOPPING
3 cups sliced summer peaches for blending	¾ cup raw almonds
2 cups sliced peaches for filling pie plate	1 cup raw walnuts
3 tablespoons fresh lemon juice	1 cup packed pitted Medjool dates (10 to 12)
1 tablespoon fresh ginger	⅛ teaspoon salt
2 tablespoons unrefined coconut oil	1 tablespoon water, if needed
1 tablespoon raw honey	1 teaspoon ground cinnamon

1. For the filling: Place the 2 cups sliced peaches in a square dish or pie plate. In a blender, combine the 3 cups of peaches, lemon juice, ginger, coconut oil, and honey and puree. Pour the puree over the 2 cups of sliced peaches.

2. For the topping: In a food processor, combine the almonds, walnuts, dates, and salt and process until the ingredients stick together. Don't over process or you will make nut butter.

3. Crumble 1½ cups of the topping over the peaches and sprinkle with the cinnamon. Chill for 3 hours. (You will have topping leftover: Add a dash of cinnamon and make Nut Tassies by rolling the topping into little balls. Chill and share!)

SERVES 8

OUR FUZZY FRIEND

Tummy troubles? Eat a peach! These babies are high in dietary fiber and water, relieving constipation. Peaches are the perfect dieter's treat, with only 38 calories in a medium peach.

Full of potassium, sodium, and calcium, peaches create glowing skin.

What happens when you are low in potassium? You are likely to have skin problems, poor memory, fatigue, anxiety, muscle weakness, hypertension, cardiac arrhythmia, congestive heart failure or heart deterioration, and vibration in your ears. Eat a peach!

When choosing peaches, always, always, always choose organic. This fruit is one of the heaviest in pesticides. By the time it arrives in your local market, the typical peach can be coated with up to nine different pesticides, according to a USDA sampling. Apples, pears, and grapes are also on the top of the charts for high pesticides.

52

KOZY SHACK CHOCOLATE PUDDING

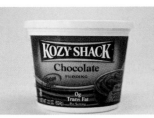

If the goal of food manufactures is to keep us hungry and craving more, they are doing an excellent job. This chocolate "flavored" dessert is filled with sugar and thickening agents, while deficient in any meaningful calories. Filling up on these "empty calories" keeps us searching the cabinets like hungry bears at a campsite. We keep putting weight on for the winter, but aren't able to shed it when the spring comes.

Avoid carrageenan. Research has shown that the popular food emulsifier (thickener) carrageenan has been linked to gastrointestinal inflammation and colon cancer. Be aware that many foods, even those certified "organic" and considered "healthy," contain carrageenan. With all good intentions, you just may be drinking your organic hemp seed milk, only to find out it contains carrageenan.

Ingredients: Low Fat Milk, Sugar, Modified Tapioca Starch, Salt, Natural Flavors, **Carrageenan**.

GOOD NEWS! AVOCADOS DON'T MAKE YOU FAT!

Of course, if you are eating avocados along with a heavily processed diet, you will pack on some pounds, but if you are eating a high-raw diet full of real food, avocados will soon become your best friend. One avocado has the ability to fill you up and keep you satisfied for hours. The avocado will stabilize your blood sugar, keeping you energized and less likely to get the munchies throughout the day. The healthy fat in the avocado is what prevents us from overeating. This is why raw desserts made with healthy fats are so extremely satisfying.

MORE GOOD NEWS!

Anandamide, which is only found in one plant—cacao—is known as the "bliss" chemical. Bottom line . . . raw chocolate makes you happy!

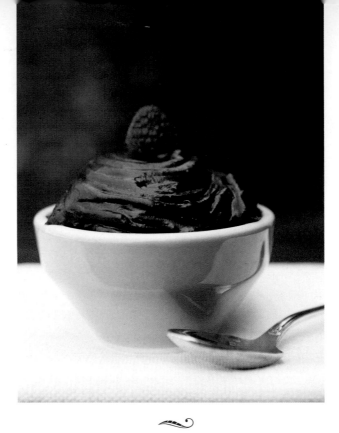

VERMONT JOE'S CHOCOLATE MOOSE

Vermont Joe's Chocolate Moose is rich in flavor, nutrition, and live enzymes. This chocolate dessert is going to keep you satisfied longer and make you less likely to devour the whole container before nightfall. This one is for Joe and all the families in Moose Country.

1½ avocados (¾ cup packed or mashed)
⅓ cup raw cacao powder, pure BLISS
¼ cup raw honey, or more to taste
¼ cup water

1 teaspoon vanilla extract
Dash of sea salt
Raspberries, for garnish

In a blender, combine the avocados, cacao powder, honey, water, vanilla, and salt and blend until smooth. Spoon into little glass dishes and top with fresh raspberries.

SERVES 4 / MAKES THE PERFECT AMOUNT
FOR TOPPING PEACE OUT CHOCOLATE CAKE
(PAGE 138)

53

YOPLAIT YOGURT

There was a time when Yoplait Yogurt was one of my very close friends. At 60 to 100 calories, "light", and in yummy flavors like Banana Cream and Key Lime Pie, I thought I'd hit a jackpot! But I never thought to ask . . . What is in this stuff?

Ingredients in Yoplait Greek Strawberry Yogurt: Cultured Pasteurized Grade A Nonfat Milk, Strawberries, Water, Sugar, contains 2% or less of: Corn Starch, Natural Flavor, Carmine (for color), Lemon Juice Concentrate, **Sucralose**, Acesulfame Potassium, Vitamin A Acetate, Vitamin D3

Sucralose, better known by its popular brand name Splenda, is one of the key ingredients that cuts the calories in "light" yogurt.

What is sucralose? Labeled by many as "natural," sucralose is anything but natural. It is an artificial sweetener made in a way that your bodies do not recognize it as food. Our bodies just want to get rid of it as quickly as possible, and that is why it becomes calorie free.

How is sucralose made? Sugar (sucrose) goes through a process that involves replacing certain parts of the sugar molecule with chlorine atoms to produce sucralose. This means sugar (sucrose) and sucralose have completely different molecular formulas, and are processed in our bodies quite differently as well.

Sucralose has a short history and there continues to be conflicting evidence regarding how much of this stuff is actually absorbed into our bodies and how toxic it is. The problem here is sucralose or Splenda is not often consumed by one-time users; we are creatures of habit, and generally find foods we like and continue to eat them often or even every day. The people eating this chemical mix consume it regularly—as I once did.

Watch out for sucralose or Splenda in these common products:

Sugar-free yogurts and ice creams

Sugar-free cookies and desserts

Sugar-free canned fruits

Sugar-free drinks (juice drinks, teas, and sodas)

Sugar-free jellies

Low-carb nutrition bars

CHA-CHA-CHIA PUDDING

If you are *not* a morning person, or seem to always be in a high-speed wobble as you are piling kids off to school, this is the fast and easy breakfast for you! This one recipe can be blended up in five minutes the day before and will last in your refrigerator for a week's worth of breakfasts. Top with blueberries, strawberries, raspberries, almonds, cashews, sunflower seeds, sliced bananas, dried cherries, and walnuts. Add a little raw honey if you like more sweetness to your morning. Sprinkle with cinnamon to taste.

1 cup raw cashews (see Note)

3 cups water

3 tablespoons Grade B maple syrup or raw honey

1 tablespoon pure vanilla extract

Pinch of salt

½ cup chia seeds

In a blender, combine the cashews, water, maple syrup, vanilla, and salt and blend until smooth and creamy. Add the chia seeds and blend lightly. Pour into a large bowl or jar and refrigerate overnight.

SERVES 9

Note: Unless you're using a high-speed blender such as a Vitamix, soak the cashews for at least 2 hours before blending. Rinse them thoroughly after soaking.

CHIA . . . NOT JUST A PET ANYMORE!

Chia absorbs up to 12 times its own weight, making you feel fuller, longer. By adding chia to your diet, you end up eating fewer calories while increasing your fiber intake. Rich in calcium: Ounce for ounce, chia seeds contain more calcium than whole milk and more omega-3 fatty acids than salmon! Omega-3's lubricate cells, keeping the reproductive system healthy. High in antioxidants, chia fights free radicals. These radicals need to be stopped! Chia is a complete protein, meaning it contains all the essential amino acids. When eaten, chia helps the body to regulate carbohydrates and the sugars they turn in to. This gives us a steady stream of energy with no crash, which is especially helpful for diabetics who are unable to process sugars properly.

54

STORE-BOUGHT CARAMEL TOPPING

Extremely high in sugar, caramel sauce provides only "empty calories" that are not going to aid your body in any way. In fact these high sugar calories actually deplete your body of nutrition. Since we only get to eat so many calories in a day, why load up on "filler foods"? Eat real food, high in nutrients and loaded with enzymes!

Ingredients: **Corn Syrup**, Sweetened Condensed Milk (**Sugar**, Water, Nonfat Milk Solids), **High Fructose Corn Syrup**, Water, Disodium Phosphate, Salt, Natural and Artificial Flavor, Caramel Color.

WICKED CARAMEL SAUCE

"Wicked" does not mean "bad" in New England parlance. "Wicked" is really, really, really good! It is so good that it is bad. Do you follow me? This is a great sauce for dipping fruit or decorating pies. Try dipping green apples and sprinkling chopped walnuts for that fall caramel apple taste.

½ cup raw cashews (see Note)
½ cup pitted Medjool dates (see Note)
½ cup raw honey or Grade B maple syrup

¼ cup water
2 teaspoons pure vanilla extract
⅛ teaspoon salt

In a blender, combine all the ingredients and blend until smooth.

Note: Unless you're using a high-speed blender such as a Vitamix, soak the cashews and dates (separately) for at least 2 hours before blending. Rinse the cashews thoroughly after soaking.

MAKES 14 (1-OUNCE) SERVINGS

GRADE B MAPLE SYRUP

This is not your Aunt Jemima's syrup. Grade B is a rich maple syrup that happens to be a fantastic supplier of energy, filled with vitamins and minerals. Unlike Grade A maple syrup, B has a very pronounced flavor. The debate is out over which has more minerals: A or B. Talk to a Vermont maple syrup sapper and you will find they won't play favorites.

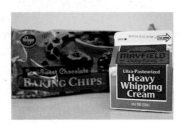

55

HOMEMADE GANACHE

Just 1 tablespoon of heavy cream has 51 calories and 5g fat, 3.5 of those coming from saturated fat. Heavy cream has no significant nutritional benefits, making it calorie-dense, yet nutrient-poor. This is a lot of wasted calories and fat.

Ingredients: Semisweet Chocolate, **Heavy Cream**, Salt

CHOCOLATE GANACHE

Let's face it: We like to cover things in chocolate! So I had to create a recipe for rich chocolate that goes on everything. This ganache is really thick and serves perfectly as a frosting for the Cioffi Bars (page 168). You can always add a bit more water for thinning out when you want the drizzle power for decorating pies or filling Mini Me's (page 160). I whip up this chocolate *bliss*, put it in a zip-seal bag, cut a tiny hole at one end, and start drizzling. I like having a bowl of Chocolate Ganache around for dipping fresh berries in when I get the inclination for a bit of decadence.

1 cup raw cacao powder	¼ cup water
½ cup raw agave nectar	½ teaspoon pure vanilla extract
⅓ cup unrefined coconut oil, warmed until softened	⅛ teaspoon salt

In a blender, combine all of the ingredient and blend until smooth and creamy. Use immediately, before ganache begins to thicken, for decorating desserts.

MAKES 13 (1-OUNCE) SERVINGS

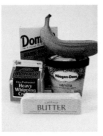

56

CLASSIC BANANAS FOSTER WITH WHIPPED CREAM

Bananas gone bad! Bananas Foster starts off with the low-calorie nutritious banana and quickly turns it into a high-calorie, high-fat, and high-sugar dessert, with ingredients added like brown sugar, butter, dark rum, banana liqueur, and vanilla ice cream. Your once fat-free banana now contains 17g of fat!

BANANA STAGES

Bananas are picked green and shipped to our markets. It's always a gamble when you stop at a local market with hopes of getting the perfect banana . . .

STAGE #1: Bananas with a lot of green are going to require some patience.

STAGE #2: Yellow bananas with tiny bits of green at the tips are firm and sweet, perfect for eating. These are good, but still not the sweetest.

STAGE #3: The perfect banana is all yellow and at its peak of freshness. This is my favorite snacking banana!

STAGE #4: The best banana for Banana Road Kill is when the yellow banana starts to get the brown sugar spots. The banana's sugar content is at its sweetest! This is also a good time to freeze your bananas to use for smoothies and ice creams.

BANANA ROAD KILL

I created Banana Road Kill with some inspiration from my little brother. He's 44 now, but as a kid, Richie always liked knock-knock jokes. Banana Road Kill is what happens when two bananas don't look both ways when they cross the road. The hardest part about this dessert is waiting for it to freeze. A little practice in patience is required here.

2 bananas, peeled
1 tablespoon raw honey

½ teaspoon cinnamon
½ cup walnuts

Let's get started:

1. Place a good 20 inches of plastic wrap on a hard surface—this could get messy. Lay the bananas on one side of the plastic wrap.

2. Fold the plastic over the bananas. Next, mash the bananas into a round banana pancake between the plastic.

3. Open the plastic wrap and drizzle on the honey (aka banana blood).

4. Next sprinkle on the cinnamon, or what I like to call the dirt.

5. Push in pieces of walnuts for gravel. (If you want to get really gross, drop in some strawberries for some strawberry guts!)

6. Freeze overnight. Break into banana bark and enjoy!

SERVES 6

> ## FEWER TEMPER TANTRUMS AND MORE SLEEP . . .
>
> Bananas contain tryptophan, serotonin, and norepinephrine—natural chemicals that supply feelings of well-being and relaxation. The B6 in bananas prevents moodiness and irritability, and promotes a restful sleep. This means a happy baby.

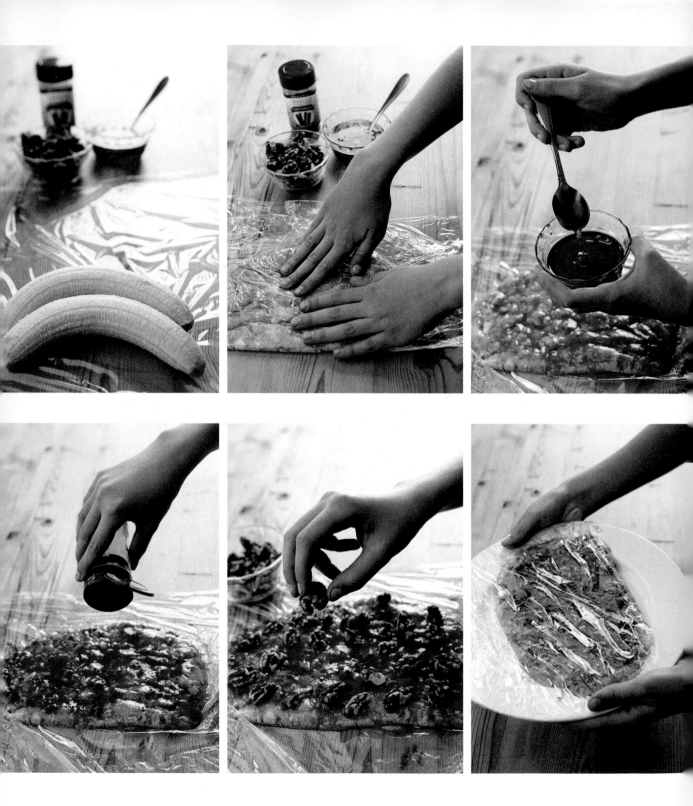

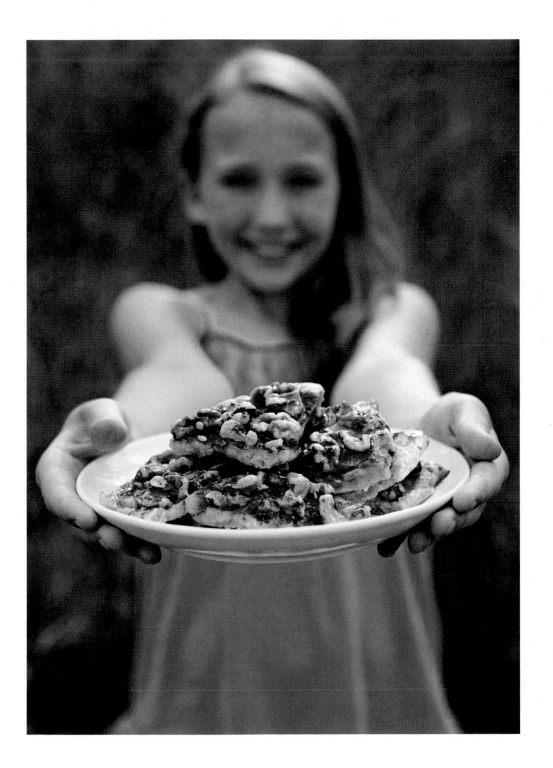

LET THEM EAT . . . DESSERT!

57

SILK VANILLA ALMOND MILK/ SO DELICIOUS COCONUT MILK BEVERAGE

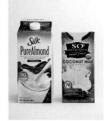

Milk sales are declining as Americans are being educated about the dangers found in the dairy industry. We just don't trust the billboards with sports figures, actors, actresses, and models flaunting those white mustaches any more. Allergies to milk are making it almost a fashion statement to be "dairy free." But what about some of the alternatives—what's in those?

Silk PureAlmond Vanilla Ingredients: Filtered Water, Almonds, Natural Evaporated Cane Juice, Calcium Carbonate, Sea Salt, Natural Vanilla Flavor, Locust Bean Gum, Gellan Gum, Sunflower Lecithin, d-alpha-Tocopherol (natural vitamin E), Zinc Gluconate, Vitamin A Palmitate, Riboflavin (B2), Vitamin B12, Vitamin D2.

SO Delicious Coconut Milk Ingredients: Organic Coconut Milk (Organic Coconut Cream, Water, Guar Gum), Organic Evaporated Cane Juice, Calcium Phosphate, Magnesium Phosphate, Carrageenan, Vitamin A Palmitate, Vitamin D2, L-Selenomethionine (Selenium), Zinc Oxide, Folic Acid, Vitamin B12.

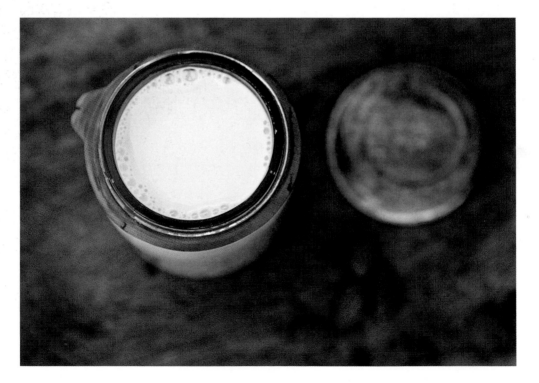

JUST ALMOND MILK

1½ cups raw almonds
6 cups clean filtered water

OPTIONAL FLAVORINGS
2 pitted Medjool dates
1 teaspoon pure vanilla extract
Pinch of salt
Dash of cinnamon

1. Soak the almonds overnight or for 12 to 14 hours. Allow enough water for your almonds to swell. (They will swell to 2 cups.)

2. Rinse the almonds and place in the blender with the 6 cups water (1:3 ratio). Blend on high until you get creamy white milk. Pour through a nut milk bag (see Note) and "milk" your almonds.

3. How to milk almonds: Line a pitcher with your nut milk bag. Pour the contents of your blender into your nut milk bag. Hold the top of the bag tight with one hand. With the other hand, start gently squeezing the almond milk through the bag. This is where I feel like I'm back on the farm milking a huge cow. There are plenty of great YouTube videos out there that will give you a great visual of both making nut milk and milking a huge cow.

4. Refrigerate the fresh almond milk in Mason jars—it will keep for a week. Shake well before pouring.

Note: Ironically, you can find the best homemade nut milk bags in the state of Vermont where the dairy cow is celebrated annually. Visit www.vt-fiddle.com.

FALL IN LOVE WITH THE ALMOND!

Almond milk is naturally low in saturated fat and has no cholesterol, with an average of 60 calories per cup. The phosphorus in almonds helps build strong teeth and bones. Almonds are one of the few proteins and one of the only nuts that are alkaline form- ing. When your body is more acidic and less alkaline, you risk osteoporosis, poor immune function, pain in the body, weight gain, and low energy.

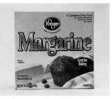

58

MRS. FIELDS® SNICKERDOODLES

Since margarine is made from vegetable oils that are chemically produced, it's not a shock to find out they contain harmful chemicals. Most vegetable oils and their products, like margarine, contain artificial antioxidants that help prevent food from spoiling too quickly. This means manufacturers can keep their products on the shelves longer.

These chemically produced oils contain residues of the chemicals and pesticides used for growing and manufacturing them. That should not come as a surprise. These chemicals have been shown to produce potential cancer-causing compounds in the body, and have also been linked to kidney/liver damage, infertility/sterility, immune problems, high cholesterol, and children behaving badly.

Ingredients: Enriched Wheat Flour (Wheat Flour, Niacin, Reduced Iron, Thiamine Mononitrate, Riboflavin, Folate), Sugar, **Margarine** [Palm Oil, Water, Salt, Whey, Monoglycerides, Soy Lecithin, Sodium Benzoate and Citric Acid (Preservatives), Artificial Flavor, Beta Carotene (Color), Vitamin A Palmitate], Fructose, Unbleached Wheat Flour.

STACY DOODLES

In talking about the healing powers of raw foods, I often start by making these cookies for potential new converts. I knew if I handed someone a shot of wheat grass, I would not get any takers. But with these fun little cookies, pretty soon I was taking orders and selling them. Stacy Doodles are hearty little cookies that pack well, replacing the typical highly processed granola and energy bars. This makes them great for kids' lunches or a hiker's backpack.

2 cups oat groats or steel-cut oats, ground into flour
1 cup raw cashews, ground into flour
¼ cup ground cinnamon (yes, ¼ *cup*)
¼ teaspoon sea salt

½ cup Grade B maple syrup
2 tablespoons unrefined coconut oil, melted until softened
1 teaspoon pure vanilla extract
¾ cup raisins

1. Set up a dehydrator.

2. In a large bowl, combine the oat flour, cashew flour, cinnamon, salt, maple syrup,

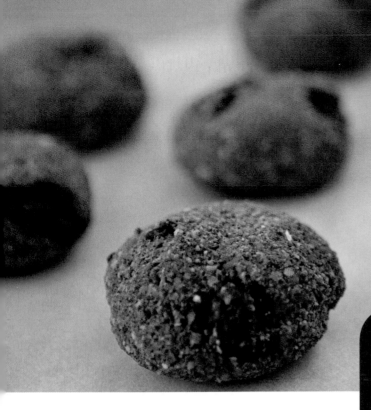

coconut oil, and vanilla. Mix well by hand. Mix in the raisins with your hands.

3. Take a chunk of dough the size of a melon ball between your hands. Work the air out and roll into little balls. Flatten into a little cookie. Add a bit more maple syrup if needed.

4. Dehydrate at 115°F for 12 hours.

MAKES ABOUT 80 TINY DOODLES

RAISINS MAKE A GREAT KIDS' SNACK!

They are:

- low in fat and cholesterol
- a good source of potassium and calcium
- high in fiber, making them ideal if your child has constipation
- made up of natural sugars, replacing the sugar-loaded snacks kids love

RAISINS ARE GREAT FOR ATHLETES!

Athletes need a lot of energy for peak performance. Many depend on glucose drinks, sports chews, and gels. These products tend to contain chemicals that end up doing the athlete more harm than good. Raisins are naturally full of glucose and fructose, supplying athletes with that added needed energy. Like all dried fruits, raisins will help in keeping weight on while exerting all this energy.

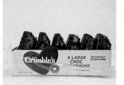

59

MRS. CRIMBLE'S MACAROONS
(plain or with chocolate)

Sugar Overload! We have five ingredients in these macaroons that are high in sugar: white sugar, coconut (assuming this is a sweetened coconut), glucose syrup, dextrose, and potato starch.

Sugar High! Have you ever gotten that "amped up" feeling after too many Skittles? Maybe you even feel a bit "buzzed."

Sugar Crash! When you consume too much sugar, your pancreas will send out the insulin for immediate sugar "clean up." Your pancreas quickly goes into overdrive trying to solve the sugar mess you just made. Pretty soon you go from sugar high to sugar crash as the pancreas keeps signaling the insulin to clean up the sugar even after the job is already done. This "sugar crash" leads us to feeling grumpy, tired, weak, and hungry . . . ironically for more sugar!

Ingredients: **Sugar**, **Coconut**, **Glucose Syrup**, Egg White, **Dextrose**, **Potato Starch**, Vegetable Oil (Palm, Palm Kernel, Coconut), Reduced Fat Cocoa Powder, Stabilizer: Sorbitan, Tristearate*, Emulsifier: Soy Lecithin.

MINI ME'S

I call these cookies Mini Me's because they are sweet, little, and blonde, like me! My mom prefers little frozen Mini Me's. Skip the dehydrating and simply pop them into the freezer.

3 to 3½ cups finely shredded unsweetened coconut, plus about 1 cup for coating
2 to 2½ cups raw cashews, ground into flour
1 cup raw honey
½ cup coconut oil, softened but not liquid

1 tablespoon fresh lemon juice
1 tablespoon pure vanilla extract
⅛ teaspoon sea salt
Shredded coconut for coating

1. Set up a dehydrator.

2. In a large bowl, combine 3 cups coconut, 2 cups cashew flour (using the smaller amount), honey, coconut oil, lemon juice, vanilla, and salt. Mix by hand. Your cookie dough should stick together but not be too wet. Mix in more cashew or coconut flour, if needed.

COCONUTS ARE AN AMAZING FOOD!

You can make so many things out of a coconut: enzyme-rich water, milk, cream, oil, butter, and dried shredded coconut. When shopping for shredded coconut, look for one that has no added sweeteners, sulfites, or preservatives, and is certified organic.

3. Take a chunk of dough the size of a melon ball between your hands. Work the air out and roll into little balls. Flatten into a puffy little cookie. Coat each cookie in shredded coconut.

4. Dehydrate at 115°F for 20 hours or until crunchy on the outside and chewy on the inside.

MAKES ABOUT 80 MINI ME'S

COCONUT OIL, FRIEND OR FOE?

Coconut has gotten a bad rap in the past for being high in saturated fat. But that's not true anymore. We are all taking a closer look at our foods in front of us. Today we are asking questions and no longer following what marketing wants us to buy. Right!?! OK, well, we are getting there for sure.

Here are some saturated FAT FACTS: Animal fats found in the meat and dairy industry contain long-chain fatty acids. Consuming too much of these long-chain fatty acids can lead to many health problems down the road, putting us at risk for obesity, heart disease, and cancer. Depending on the individual, some of us are more susceptible than others to these diseases. Don't risk it!

Coconut fats consist mostly of medium-chain fatty acids. These medium-chain fatty acids are easily metabolized by the body and convert quickly into energy; they actually help strengthen our immune system and protect us from heart disease.

VARIATION: MINI ME'S MEETS CHOCOLATE GANACHE

The Mini Me's (page 160) really play well with chocolate. A very simple way to dress this little cookie up is to fill them with Chocolate Ganache (page 150). The flavors come together in pure joy! Create a small thumbprint in the center of each Mini Me's before dehydrating. Fill a pastry bag or a small plastic sandwich bag with the Chocolate Ganache. (Be sure to make the Chocolate Ganache right before using as it thickens as it sits. If it gets too thick, thin it out with a little water.) Cut a tiny hole in the tip of the plastic bag and fill the centers of the dehydrated Mini Me's. Refrigerate.

Note: Dehydrate Mini Me's first, then fill with Chocolate Ganache.

CAFFEINE?

Contrary to the rumors, raw chocolate (cacao) does not contain caffeine. Raw chocolate contains theobromine, which is a relative of caffeine but not a nervous system stimulant. Theobromine dilates the blood vessels that are part of the cardiovascular system, making the heart's job easier.

Personally, when I consume raw chocolate in small doses on a regular basis, I feel creative, inspired, and focused. Nothing can bring me down on chocolate—I thank chocolate for my best work!

I never feel a high on cacao; nor do I feel that all too common low I once felt after having caffeine. However, I never have cacao in the evenings; raw chocolate can be a stimulant for some and affect people's ability to sleep. Everybody reacts differently to chocolate. See what works for you!

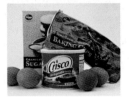

60

HOMEMADE SARAH BERNHARDT COOKIE

Sarah Bernhardt was a famous French actress in the late 19th century. Apparently while touring Amsterdam, she sampled and fell in love with this chocolate-covered macaroon. The owner of the shop was so honored, he named the little confection after her.

Ingredients: Sugar, Semisweet Chocolate, Eggs, Almond Paste, Vegetable Shortening, Water, Almond Extract, Salt.

~~

SARAH BERNHARDT COOKIE, GONE RAW!

Re-creating by upgrading . . . . I often take whatever ingredients are used in a recipe and simply "upgrade" them to a healthier level. That is fairly simple with these delicious little "Bernhardts." Here are a few examples of the types of change I make:

Instead of sugar, use raw honey.

Instead of semisweet (processed) chocolate, use raw chocolate (cacao).

Instead of all the fat coming from eggs and vegetable shortening, use unrefined coconut oil.

Instead of almond paste, use raw nuts.

Instead of baking, dehydrate!

1. Mini Me's Meet Chocolate Ganache (page 150)

2. Hard Chocolate Coating (page 166), melted

3. Make ganache-filled Mini Me's as directed. Freeze your cookies for super firmness. Now you are ready for dipping!

4. Dip each cookie into the melted chocolate coating. Place the cookies on wax paper or nonstick liners for easy removal. Chill.

MAKES APPROXIMATELY 18 COOKIES

EAT RAW, NOT COOKED

IT'S TIME TO RECONNECT WITH CHOCOLATE...

The chocolate most people eat today is a highly processed chocolate. All the nutritional benefits have been destroyed by fire and then filled with added sugar, milk fats, saturated fats, and corn syrup. While raw chocolate can be a potent and beneficial medicine, processed chocolate can actually promote heart disease, high cholesterol, high blood pressure, and weight gain. Eat raw chocolate, not cooked!

61

SNICKERS® BAR

"Snickers satisfies you!"

This was the jingle I grew up hearing on TV. If I was hungry, I was told to reach for a Snickers. I really did believe in my young mind that Snickers was a good-for-you energy bar, and it was all fun and games until I became a teenager and decided I didn't want to be that chubby kid any more.

Why is candy not a good snack food for kids?

Let's say kids need to consume 1,200 calories a day. Eating a Snickers bar at 280 calories either gives them way too many calories, or they end up forfeiting much healthier snacks that would provide more nutrients and staying power.

Should kids never have candy? That sounds painfully sad. We just need to "upgrade" our candy choices. With all the cookie/bar/candy recipes in this section, you will have plenty of options to play with. Enjoy!

Ingredients: Milk Chocolate (Sugar, Cocoa Butter, Chocolate, Skim Milk, Lactose, Milkfat, Soy Lecithin, Artificial Flavor), Peanuts, Corn Syrup, Sugar, Milkfat, Skim Milk, Partially Hydrogenated Soybean Oil, Lactose, Salt, Egg Whites, Chocolate, Artificial Flavor.

~~~

HARD CHOCOLATE COATING

. . . for Chocolate-Covered Everything!

If you don't have a double boiler you can improvise one by placing a glass or stainless steel bowl over a pot of simmering water.

1 cup raw cacao paste, shaved for easy melting ⅛ teaspoon sea salt
¼ cup raw honey

1. In the top of a double boiler, gently melt the cacao shavings over a pan of simmering water, stirring constantly. Stir in the honey and salt.

2. Before the chocolate is completely melted, remove from the heat and continue to stir while the chocolate continues to melt. Warning: There is a point of no return if

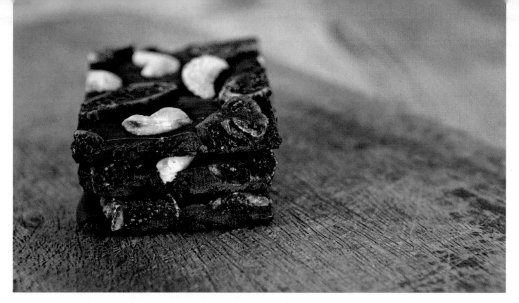

you overheat your chocolate. Simply warm until most of the chocolate is melted. Do not cook your chocolate. It can get very ugly, very quickly. Trust me.

3. Begin dipping and coating *everything* in chocolate.

VARIATION: CASHEW & FIG CHOCOLATE BARK

Pour the melted chocolate out onto a nonstick dehydrator sheet (for easy removal). Add raw cashews and chopped figs to the melted chocolate. Chill in the refrigerator. Cut into candy bars.

MAKES 6 CANDY BARS

QUICK SNACK

With kids' hectic schedules these days, it's all too easy to head to the closest vending machine for a quick pick-me-up. But dried fruit and raw nuts make for a perfect combination and an easy energy source when you're on the go. Figs are rich in calcium, making for stronger bones and teeth. Raw cashews have a high energy density and a high amount of dietary fiber, which makes them great for weight management. And raw cacao contains more vitamin C than any other food in the world (not found in processed chocolate). The high heat has destroyed all nutrients, leaving this once powerful food *dead.*

62

HOMEMADE EAGLE BRAND® MAGIC COOKIE BARS

These five-layer cookie bars debuted in the 1960s, and have continued to be Eagle Brand condensed milk's most popular recipe, becoming a tradition for many families around our country.

What's in this beloved treat? The recipe is loaded with refined sugar! When we consume refined sugars our bodies have to produce a rush of insulin to help metabolize this sugar. We soon feel that "sugar crash," leading us to reach for that second and third bar. Pretty soon, the whole pan is gone! This in turn can lead to packing on the excess weight, especially around holidays when sugar is in abundance.

Ingredients: Graham Cracker Crumbs, Butter, Eagle Brand Sweetened Condensed Milk, Semi-sweet Chocolate Chips, Flaked Coconut, Chopped Nuts.

CIOFFI BARS

The Cioffi family is a family of foodies. Phil and Debbie Cioffi have a collection of old-favorite family recipes, all of them very rich in traditional ingredients. I asked them for a challenge: Give me your very favorite recipe and I will turn it into a guilt-free treat that will continue to satisfy the whole family.

They did not have to think long. The "Magic Bar"! This buttery graham cracker crust topped with chocolate, nuts, and coconut was first introduced to Phil by his mom in the 1960s. And the recipe for it is still easily found on the label of a sweetened condensed milk can today. I have re-created the recipe and turned it into something much healthier. Thank you, Phil and Debbie Cioffi, for your inspiration.

CRUST	TOPPINGS
2 cups raw walnuts	Wicked Caramel Sauce (page 148)
1 cup Medjool dates	Chocolate Ganache (page 160)
½ cup raw coconut palm sugar	⅓ cup chopped walnuts
½ cup unsweetened shredded coconut	⅓ cup unsweetened shredded coconut
⅛ teaspoon salt	

1. For the crust: In a food processor, combine all the ingredients and process until the ingredients stick together. Don't overprocess or you will make nut butter. Press the crust firmly into the bottom of a 9 x 11-inch baking dish. Put in the freezer so the crust is firm before adding your next layer.

2. Meanwhile, make the Wicked Caramel Sauce.

3. Spread a thin layer of the caramel over the frozen crust. (Keep the extra sauce for dipping apples. The kids will love it!) Return to the freezer until the caramel layer hardens.

4. Meanwhile, make the Chocolate Ganache. Layer the chocolate on top of the hardened caramel layer.

5. Decorate with raw walnut pieces and organic dried shredded unsweetened coconut. Refrigerate. These bars will keep for a couple of weeks in the refrigerator.

SERVINGS: 30

COCONUT PALM SUGAR, WHERE HAVE YOU BEEN ALL MY LIFE!

To re-create the flavor of my Cioffi Family's graham cracker crust, I needed the right sugar, and along came coconut palm sugar, which is a completely natural, unrefined sugar coming from the flowers growing high on top of coconut trees. This sugar is low-glycemic (meaning no sugar crash) and rich in key phytonutrients, vitamins, and minerals, including potassium, iron, zinc, and vitamins B1, B2, B3, and B6.

Most sweeteners are highly refined, or bleached, like white table sugar. Not coconut palm sugar! You get it just as it comes, a nice warm rich brown color, tasting amazingly like brown sugar with hints of butterscotch and caramel.

63

HOMEMADE FUDGE

During the holidays, fudge seems to become a major food group. Fudge lines dessert trays at parties nationwide, and gifts of fudge are beautifully wrapped in shiny bows during this festive season. Just for today, let's "unwrap" this ever-popular holiday treat.

The most common fudge ingredients include sugar, semisweet chocolate chips, margarine or butter, vanilla, evaporated milk, nuts, marshmallows (or marshmallow crème). From See's Candies to Grandma's homemade fudge, marshmallows are consistently a key fudge ingredient. Most marshmallows and marshmallow cremes are made of corn syrup, even more sugar, chemicals, preservatives, artificial flavor, and color. Our bodies are not meant to eat all these chemicals, preservatives, fake flavors, and food dyes. Now if you are going to only be indulging in a single piece of fudge during a holiday party, you will be fine. But let's be honest, the holidays bring a daily banquet of these not-so-healthy treats.

Don't be discouraged. I have for you an excellent raw fudge your guests will absolutely love!

ANTIOXIDANTS AND CHOCOLATE

Our bodies are in a constant fight against infection and diseases. Normal body functions like breathing and exercise naturally produce free radicals, but we start to accumulate excess free radicals from doing things like tanning, smoking, and alcohol consumption. These free radicals attack healthy cells, which makes us more susceptible to cancer and heart disease. Free radicals can also weaken our immune system. Antioxidants help us to strengthen our immune system, making us more capable of warding off colds and flus. How do we fight off the free radicals and get more antioxidants? First of all, if you are smoking or tanning, quit ASAP and eat more chocolate!

Raw chocolate (cacao) is a free radical shield. It contains the highest concentration of antioxidants of any food in the world. This is the big news I have been waiting for all my life! By weight, raw chocolate has more antioxidants than red wine and blueberries combined. Sadly, most chocolate we find on the grocery shelves are heavily processed and refined, giving none of these medicinal benefits.

Allergies to raw unprocessed chocolate are rare. Typically the person is allergic to milk or dairy products used in chocolate products. Some people can be allergic to processed chocolate but not allergic to raw cacao.

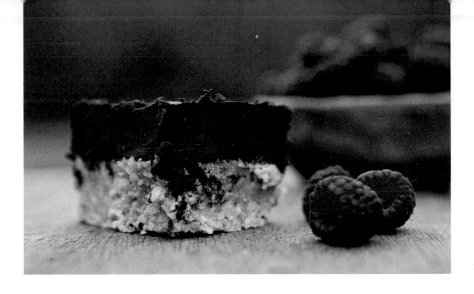

CHOCOLATE MACAROON FUDGE BARS

As I am packing up from my week with my De'Alio Family, and loading my car for the next week's journey, Kimmie begs me for one more rich chocolatey treat to keep her supplied through the holidays ahead. In minutes, I whip up a surprise new creation. Even I was shocked at how delicious it was! This recipe has not changed one ingredient since that morning I made it for my new friend. I love you Gary, Kimmie, Drew, Alec, and Wes. Here's to you!

MACAROON LAYER

3 cups finely shredded coconut

2 cups raw cashews, ground into flour

½ cup raw honey

¼ cup unrefined coconut oil, softened but not liquid

1 tablespoon pure vanilla extract

¼ teaspoon sea salt

FUDGE LAYER

2 cups raw cacao powder

1 cup raw agave nectar

⅔ cup unrefined coconut oil

¼ teaspoon salt

1. **For the macaroon layer:** In a food processor, combine all the ingredients and process.

2. Pat the mixture into a 9 x 11-inch glass baking dish or square "brownie pan." Chill.

3. **For the fudge layer:** In a food processor, combine all the ingredients and process until blended. Frost the macaroon layer with this chocolate fudge layer. Chill.

MAKES ABOUT 30 BARS

LET THEM EAT . . . DESSERT!

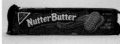

64

NABISCO NUTTERBUTTER PEANUT BUTTER SANDWICH COOKIES

Hydrogenated oil for kids. . . . If you want a kid who is hyper, chubby, and irritable, feed them hydrogenated oils and vegetable shortenings. These are some pretty evil oils considered to be "trans fats." Manufacturers created these trans fats via a process called hydrogenation. Hydrogenation is when vegetable oils are turned into solid fats by adding hydrogen atoms. Why would anyone do that? This creates food that can stay on the shelves for a long time. These trans fats are lurking everywhere in a long list of foods including crackers, chips, cereals, candies, cookies, snack foods, salad dressings, fried foods, margarine, and vegetable shortening.

Ingredients: Enriched Flour (Wheat Flour, Niacin, Reduced Iron, Thiamine Mononitrate [Vitamin B1], Riboflavin [Vitamin B2], Folic Acid), Sugar, Peanut Butter (Peanuts, Corn Syrup Solids, Hydrogenated Rapeseed and/or Cottonseed and/or Soybean Oils, Salt), Soybean Oil and/or Palm Oil, High Fructose Corn Syrup, Graham Flour (Whole Grain Wheat Flour), Partially Hydrogenated Cottonseed Oil, Salt, Leavening (Baking Soda and/or Calcium Phosphate), Cornstarch, Soy Lecithin (Emulsifier), Vanillin-An Artificial Flavor.

"PEANUT BUTTER" FREEZER COOKIES

These are simple cookies that can be made with your kids. There is no baking or dehydrating needed. "Peanut Butter" Freezer Cookies are great for kids allergic to peanuts, since no peanuts are harmed in the making of these little treats!

½ cup raw almond butter
¼ cup raw honey
1 teaspoon pure vanilla extract

⅛ teaspoon salt
2 cups raw cashews, ground into flour

1. In a bowl, combine the almond butter, honey, vanilla, and salt and mix by hand. Add the cashew flour and mix until you get a firm cookie dough consistency.

2. Roll the dough into little balls the size of a melon ball (I like little cookies. They are cute. Big cookies are not.) Flatten the cookies with a fork. Freeze for a couple of hours. Store these cookies in the freezer.

MAKES ABOUT 52 LITTLE COOKIES

EAT RAW, NOT COOKED

ALMOND BUTTER VS. PEANUT BUTTER

• With more than twice the magnesium, almond butter wins as the better bone builder.

• Almonds have double the fiber of the peanut, 86% more iron, and 169% more vitamin E. Score for the almond!

• For cell repair, almond butter reigns with higher phosphorus.

• For the grand slam, almonds smash the peanuts in a big win with three times more calcium!

VARIATION: "PEANUT BUTTER" CUPS

Dip these little frozen cookies in melted Hard Chocolate Coating (page 166) for a great alternative to peanut butter cups. Chill.

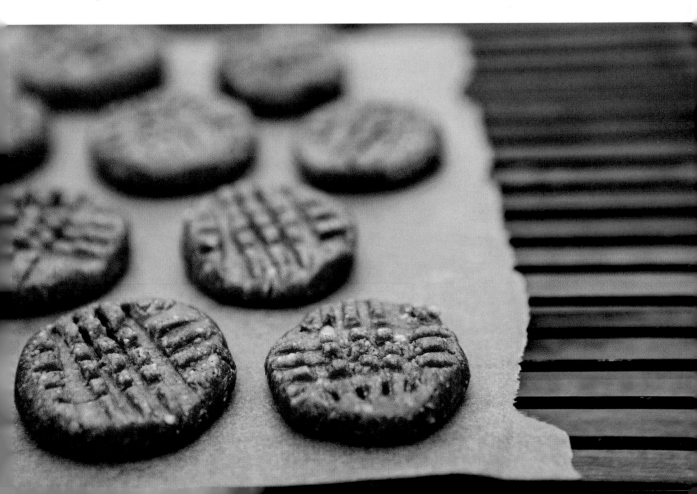

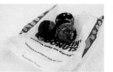

65

DUNKIN DONUTS® CHOCOLATE MUNCHKINS

"America runs on Dunkin." Half of us in America have been projected to be obese by 2030. This means more diabetes, more heart disease, more strokes, and more cancer. With ingredients like these, I don't think this projection is far off.

CONTAINS ALLERGENS: Eggs, Milk, Soy, Wheat.

INGREDIENTS: Munchkin: Enriched Bleached Wheat Flour (Wheat Flour, Malted Barley Flour, Niacin, Reduced Iron, Thiamin Mononitrate, Enzyme, Riboflavin, Folic Acid), Palm Oil, Water, Sugar, Skim Milk, Soybean Oil, Cocoa processed with alkali, contains less than 2% of the following: Leavening (Baking Soda, Sodium Acid Pyrophosphate, Sodium Aluminum Phosphate, Monocalcium Phosphate), Egg Whites, Whey (a milk derivative), Salt, Artificial Flavor, Sodium Caseinate (a milk derivative), Soy Flour, Modified Corn Starch, Defatted Soy Flour, Soy Protein Isolate, Wheat Starch, Polyglycerol Esters of Fatty Acids, Guar Gum, Carbohydrate Gum, Soy Lecithin, Gelatinized Wheat Starch, Xanthan Gum, Cellulose Gum, L-Cysteine Hydrochloride; Glaze: Sugar, Water, Maltodextrin, Contains 2% or less of: Mono and Diglycerides, Agar, Cellulose Gum, Citric Acid, Potassium Sorbate (Preservative), Artificial Flavor.

CHOCOLATE DONUT HOLES

1½ cups raw walnuts
1 cup packed pitted Medjool dates (10 to 12)
⅓ cup raw cacao powder

1 teaspoon pure vanilla extract
⅛ teaspoon salt
1 tablespoon water, if needed

In a food processor, combine the walnuts, dates, cacao powder, vanilla, and salt and process until mixture the sticks together. Add a tiny amount of water if needed to moisten the mixture. Don't overprocess or you will make nut butter. Take about 1 heaping tablespoon of the mixture in your hands and press together. Work the air out. Roll into little balls and chill.

MAKES ABOUT 24 DONUT HOLES

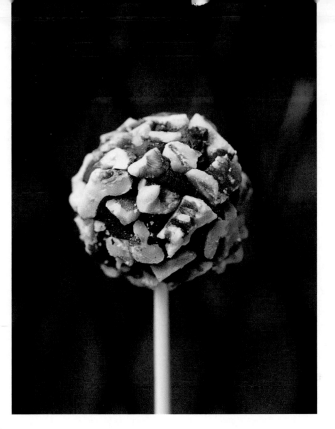

VARIATION: DONUT HOLE CAKE POPS

Before chilling the donut holes, insert pop sticks (you'll need about 18). Meanwhile, make the Hard Chocolate Coating (page 166). Dip the pops in the melted chocolate. Sprinkle on chopped walnut pieces and set aside in the refrigerator for the chocolate to set. While a Styrofoam square works great for standing your pops up as they harden, I have found standing your pops up in a banana works as well. Makes about 18 cake pops.

CHOCOLATE TOOTHPASTE?

As it turns out, there is something in raw cacao that fights tooth decay. Specifically, the husk of the unprocessed raw chocolate bean is what possesses an antibacterial effect in the mouth, and effectively fights against plaque. Chocolate has been found to be much less harmful than many other sweet treats because the antibacterial agents in raw cacao beans offset the high sugar levels in desserts.

HOMEMADE OREO® TRUFFLES

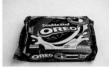

Since the introduction of the Oreo in 1912, this cookie has gone on to be the best-selling cookie in the United States. Growing up, the Oreo was definitely a staple in our home, since this was my dad's very favorite cookie. We all had our Oreo eating technique. I was a "dunker," and my little brother was a "pull them apart and eat the creamer." I don't think we ever looked at or cared about what was actually in an Oreo. Let's find out today:

Ingredients: Sugar, Enriched Flour (Wheat Flour, Niacin, Reduced Iron, Thiamine Mononitrate {Vitamin B1}, Riboflavin {Vitamin B2}, Folic Acid), High Oleic Canola Oil and/or Palm Oil and/or Canola Oil, and/or Soybean Oil, Cocoa (Processed with Alkali), **High Fructose Corn Syrup**, Cornstarch, Leavening (Baking Soda and/or Calcium Phosphate), Salt, Soy Lecithin (Emulsifier), Vanill-N—An Artificial Flavor, Chocolate.

High fructose corn syrup is commonly used in processed foods in the place of sugar. It is present in almost everything from cookies and sodas to your kid's ketchup. This sugar substitute is used because it is cheaper than sugar. High fructose corn syrup is harder for your body to digest than natural sugars. Be gentle to your body. When you need a sweet treat, choose a natural sugar, like fruit, dried fruit, or raw honey.

EAT RAW, NOT COOKED . . . CHOCOLATE

The benefits of raw chocolate are most rewarding to me. I get to feel good about indulging in something I love . . . chocolate! The benefits just seem too good to be true; from cavity prevention to weight management to fighting free radicals to a mood enhancer, raw chocolate is the bomb!

With all these medicinal qualities available to you in raw chocolate, it is important to understand one thing: When you cook or process raw chocolate, the fat in the chocolate turns into a "trans fat." This can cause and inflammatory reaction. In addition, dairy products and sugars don't make the situation any better. Always remember, when it comes to getting the most out of your chocolate, eat raw, not cooked.

TRUFFLES FOR SUE

Sue loves chocolate and I love Sue. These are for Sue. After creating these Truffles for Sue, I have incorporated them into every dinner party since. When guests arrive, they are greeted with truffles. What better way to get a party started than with joy created by raw chocolate!

⅓ cup raw coconut butter
½ cup raw honey
1 cup raw cacao powder

⅛ teaspoon salt
For coating: raw cacao powder or finely shredded unsweetened coconut

In a food processor, combine all the ingredients and process until you get a nice creamy mound of chocolate. Chill the mixture in the refrigerator for about 20 minutes or until firm. Roll into small balls the size of a melon ball. Dip in cacao powder or finely shredded coconut. Chill.

MAKES ABOUT 24 TRUFFLES

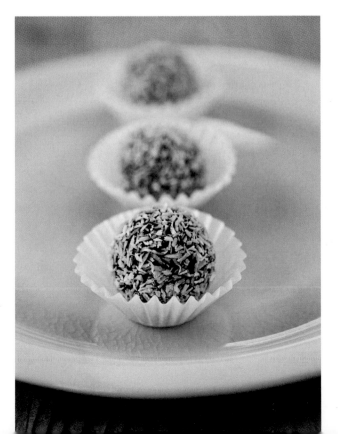

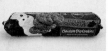

PILLSBURY® CHOCOLATE CHIP FLAVORED COOKIES

My only experience with baking has been with Pillsbury Chocolate Chip slice and bake cookies. Why would you bake any other way? They are easy, yummy, and no clean-up! Let's find out what makes these cookies so yummy:

Ingredients: Flour Bleached Enriched (Wheat Flour, Niacin, Ferrous Sulfate, Thiamine Mononitrate (Vitamin B1), Riboflavin (Vitamin B2), Folic Acid (Vitamin B9)), Sugar, **Flavored Chips Chocolate** (Sugar, Palm Kernel Oil Partially Hydrogenated, Cocoa, Cocoa Processed with Alkali, Dextrose, Soy Lecithin), Soybean(s) Oil Partially Hydrogenated and, Cottonseed Oil, Water, contains 2% or less of the Following: (Molasses, Wheat Protein Isolate, Baking Powder (Baking Soda, Sodium Aluminum Phosphate), Salt, Egg(s), Flavor(s) Artificial, Milk Non-Fat

What are artificial flavors? Once foods go through the intense process of creating a convenience product, much of the original flavor is destroyed. So scientists and chemicals have joined forces in a lab to transfuse flavor back into these foodlike products. Thus, "artificial" flavors are born.

What about "natural" flavors? What if the package says it contains "natural flavors"? These words may make you feel better while eating it, but this simply means that something not natural was done to something natural. Unlike artificial flavors, natural flavors actually do start out from natural foods like spices, fruit, and poultry. They are then transformed into chemical additives.

~~~

CHOCOLATE CHIP COOKIE DOUGH BALLS

Every family I feed always ends up getting its very own recipe. So when the best book people in town at Simon & Schuster and Gallery Books decided to adopt me, I went to work creating for them their very own recipe. This one had to be GREAT! Thank you all for taking a chance on me, and for letting me feed you. Love, S

(P.S. These treats taste so much like cookie dough, I am afraid someone may try baking them. Don't.)

1½ cups oat groats or steel-cut oats, ground into flour

3 cups raw cashews, ground into flour

1 teaspoon salt

½ cup soft raw honey (see Note)

1 teaspoon pure vanilla extract

1 tablespoon water, if needed

Truffles for Sue (page 177)

½ cup raw cacao powder, for coating

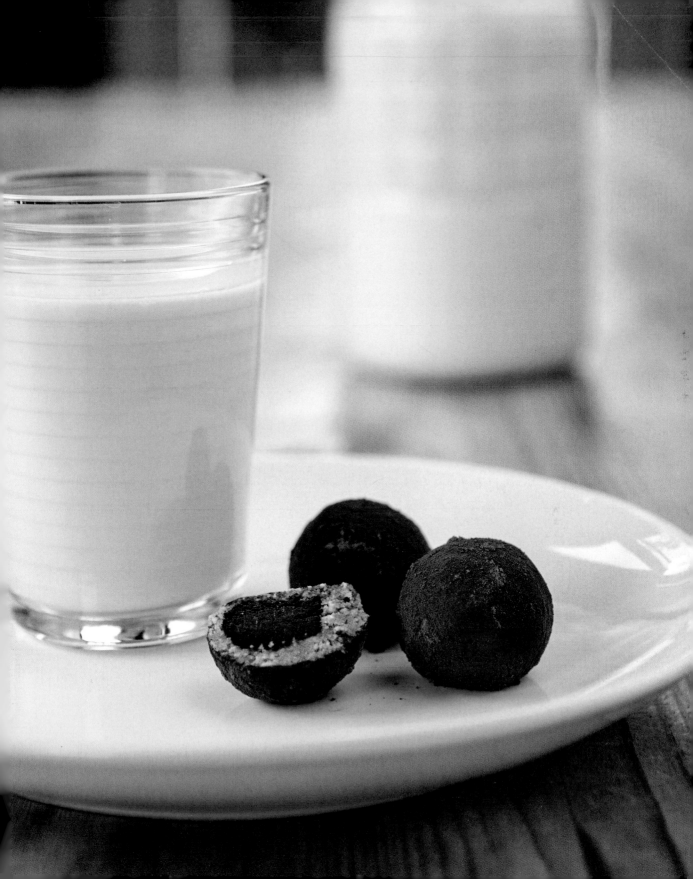

10 REASONS TO TAKE RAW CHOCOLATE TO THE OFFICE

1. Magnesium supports brain power.

2. Phenylethylamine (PEA) makes us alert and focused.

3. The anandamides in chocolate: We get our best work done when we are blissed out on endorphins!

4. Tryptophan elevates the mood.

5. Serotonin alleviates stress.

6. Zinc supports the immune system.

7. Vitamin C wards off the common cold.

8. Omega-6 fatty acids prevent "brain fog."

9. Chromium helps balance blood sugar.

10. Manganese oxygenates the blood.

AND ONE MORE FOR GOOD MEASURE . . .

11. Fiber . . . let's face it: We are all a lot happier when our bowels are moving.

1. In a large bowl, mix together the oat flour, cashew flour, and salt. Knead in the honey and vanilla by hand. The cookie dough should stick together but not be too wet. If too dry, add the water. If too wet, add additional oat or cashew flour.

2. Take about 1 tablespoon of the dough between your hands and work the air out. Roll into little balls and flatten, creating a little "hammock" to fill in with a tiny chocolate truffle.

3. Make the truffles, forming them into tiny little ½-teaspoon-size balls. Fill the inside of each cookie dough ball with a truffle. Fold the dough around the truffle and roll into a ball. Roll in the cacao powder. Chill.

MAKES 45 TO 50 COOKIES

Note: Some raw honeys are very hard. You will want a soft raw honey, making it easier to knead into the dough.

VARIATION: JIMMY CHEWS

Jimmy Chews evolved naturally from the Chocolate Chip Cookie Dough recipe when Fireman Jimmy suggested replacing the chocolate center with a chewy center. What a fabulous idea, Jimmy! Make the dough from Chocolate Chip Cookie Dough Balls (page 178) and shape as directed. But instead of a truffle, fill the center of each cookie with a few dried cherries (you'll need about ½ cup). Then close up and roll in ½ cup raw coconut palm sugar to coat. Chill.

CHERRY BOMB

Cherries are natural sources for melatonin, the chemical that regulates sleep. Jimmy will be able to adjust his sleep after coming off his shift at the firehouse. And no more jet lag for me! Dried cherries, fresh cherries, and tart cherry juice (the tart cherry juice will have less sugar) are all three great natural sleep aids. Pack cherries for your next flight and eat them an hour before you want to get some sleep. After arriving in your new time zone, eat cherries each night before bed for three nights in a row . . . ZZZZZZZZZZ.

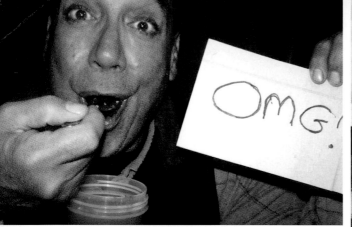
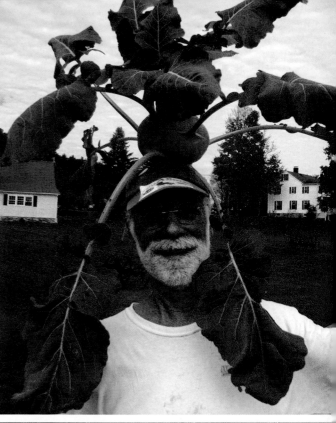
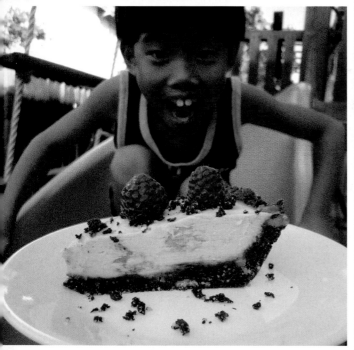
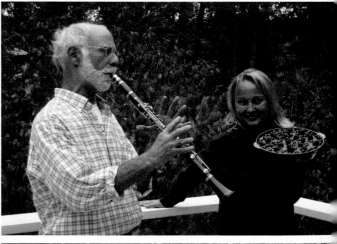
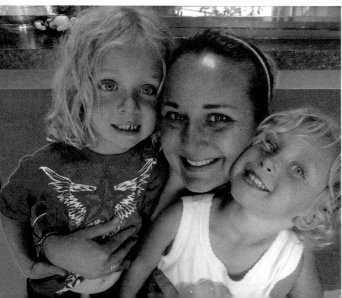
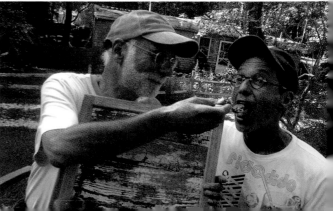

Epilogue

Testimonials

The greatest blessing in life is to have the love of family. These are just a few of my families that feed my soul, and who are my co-creators and inspirations for *Eat Raw, Not Cooked*.

❧

"Having Stacy stay with us for a week changed our lives! As a family of five with three boys (ages 18, 16, and 11), we are always on the go! Learning how to make the best choices in ingredients and finding fun and delicious ways to nourish ourselves is no easy feat. The ripple effect that Stacy so lovingly created will last forever! You see, it's not just the recipes that make this book special . . . it's Stacy herself!"

—Kimberly D'Alelio, Boston, MA

❧

"Where do I start with Stacy? She is a wonderful and courageous woman whose passion for raw foods enchants and entrances every person she encounters. If you get a chance to have Stacy come into your home for a week, please do not pass it up. It will change your life completely. She can work wonders in any kitchen, and she can make anyone into a raw food chef in just a few short days. Her time with me was priceless, and I look forward to having her return soon for another visit."

—Michael West, Vineyard Haven, MA

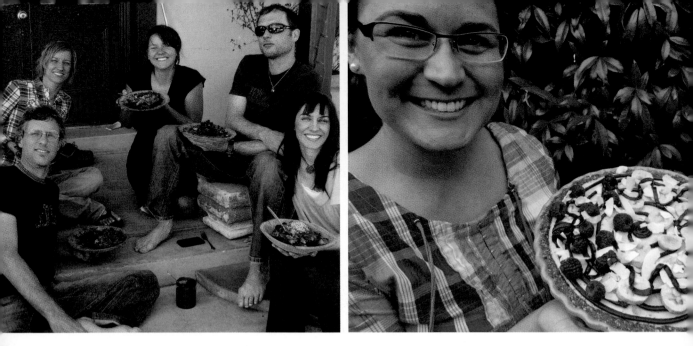

"Stacy, I love your warmhearted approach to raw foods. I know the Sunny Slope Farm Soup is not raw, but when I am eating more raw foods, it sure hits the spot! Thank you."
—Sharon Strimling, Oak Bluffs, MA

"Dear Stacy, we have made your delicious spring rolls with the amazing peanut sauce dozens of times. The kids love to make them with their friends when they are over playing. Hope all is well with you. We continue getting healthier and stronger. Thanks for everything. Lots of love!"
—Kathleen Peterson, San Diego, CA

"Thanks to 'Chips' & Dip, our seven-year-old will now eat romaine. Stacy Stowers, you are definitely known as the 'Vegetable Whisperer' at our house!"
—Johnny Shui, Fremont, CA

Epilogue

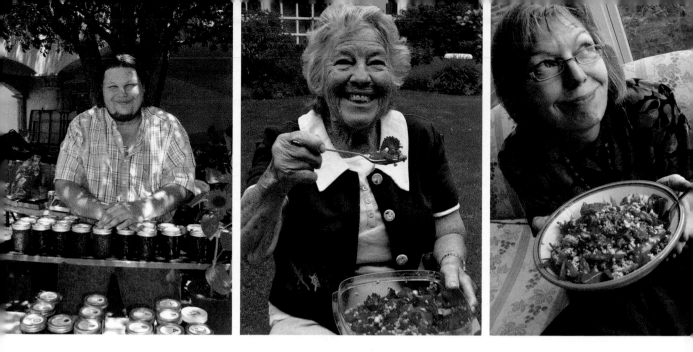

"As Firemen, our job involves seeing people on the worst day of their lives.
Thank you for bringing us the Happy Shake!"
—Chief Shivers, Forsyth County Fire Department

"The Key Lime Pie is now our department's preworkout food."
—Shane Smith, San Ramone Fire Department, San Ramone, CA

"In the Fire Department, eating was just something that got in the way,
now food is part of our wellness. Thank you Stacy Stowers!"
—John Payne, Glendale Fire Department, Glendale, CA

Epilogue

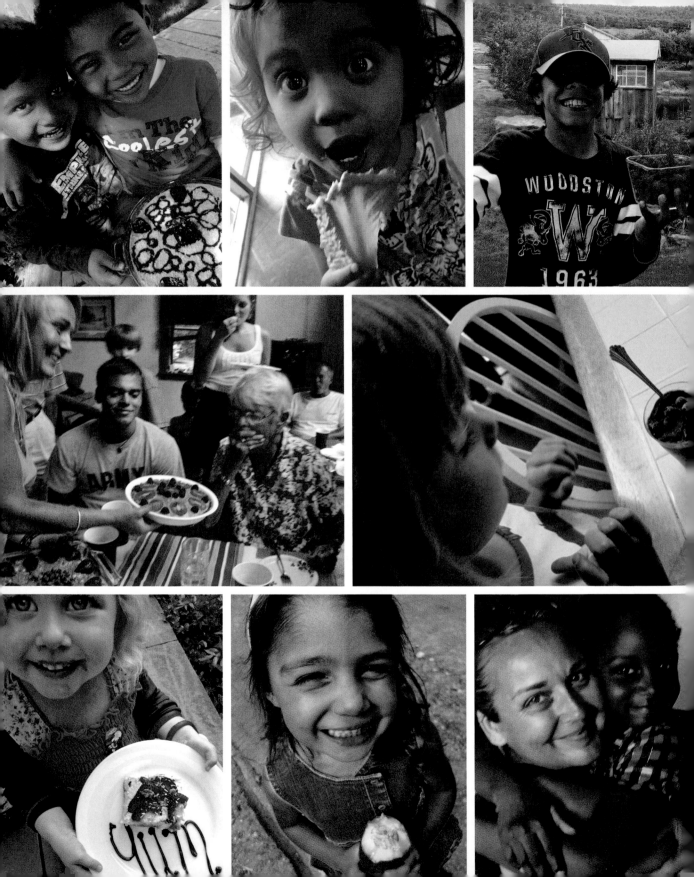

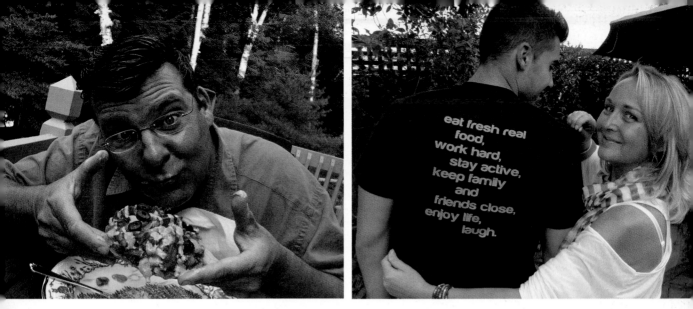

On shirt: eat fresh real food, work hard, stay active, keep family and friends close, enjoy life, laugh.

＊

"Good Morning Weed Hopper! After going for my checkup I thought I would send you a line. My doctor is one of the top cardio doctors in the country and I got him doing the Happy Shakes! He told me how tired he was and how healthy I looked. So I faxed him over your recipe. I feel like I'm 18 again and I have the whole office eating Happy Shakes! Stay warm & take care . . . THANK YOU STACY!!!!!! You got me on the right track."

—David, Long Beach, CA

＊

"Stacy, I don't know what it is about you, but I think you create joy! I had my Happy Shake this morning and I'm making the Broccoli Alfredo again tonight. Thank you!"

—Kelly McCoy, Greenwich, CT

＊

"You don't have to step out of your life to eat raw."

—The Husband, New York, NY

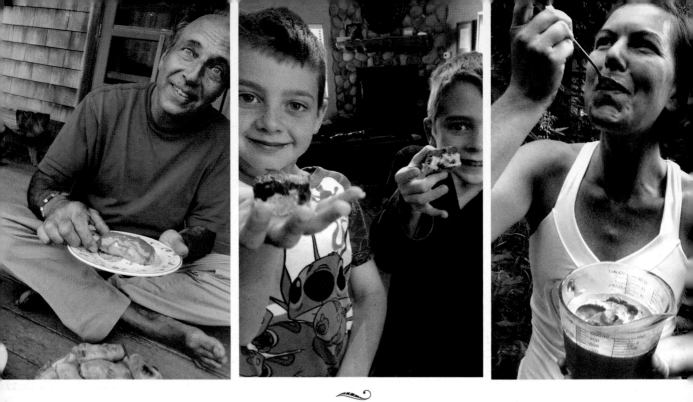

"I can do this! You have taught me to love veggies of all sorts and not be afraid of what different combos could taste like. I love everything I eat now. And what I love even more is that my kids love it, too. Thank you so so much!!!"
—Jean-Marie, Ventura, CA

ARE YOU READY?
(inspired by a rainy day Happy Shake)

"Today. Today is a good day. Rain, dark clouds.
Heavy rains; nourishing. Liquid base.
It could be water. Not bitter. Glorious heavenly Happy
Shake. Feeling now the brightness heavenly Happy
Shake. The child in me is dancing. I am hugging every
tree. I'm in love. Are you ready?"
—Mark Halperin, Dover, MA

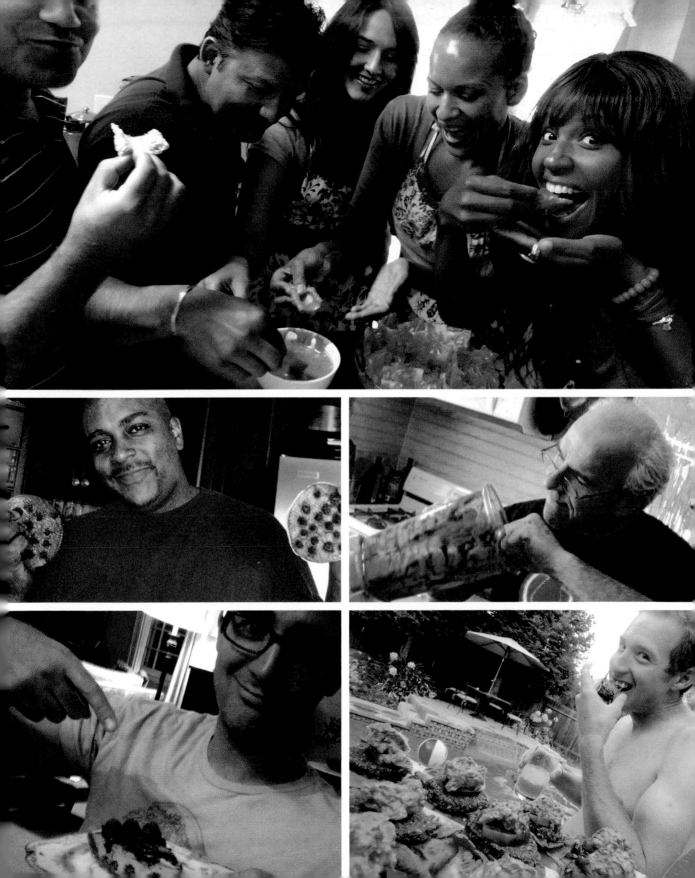

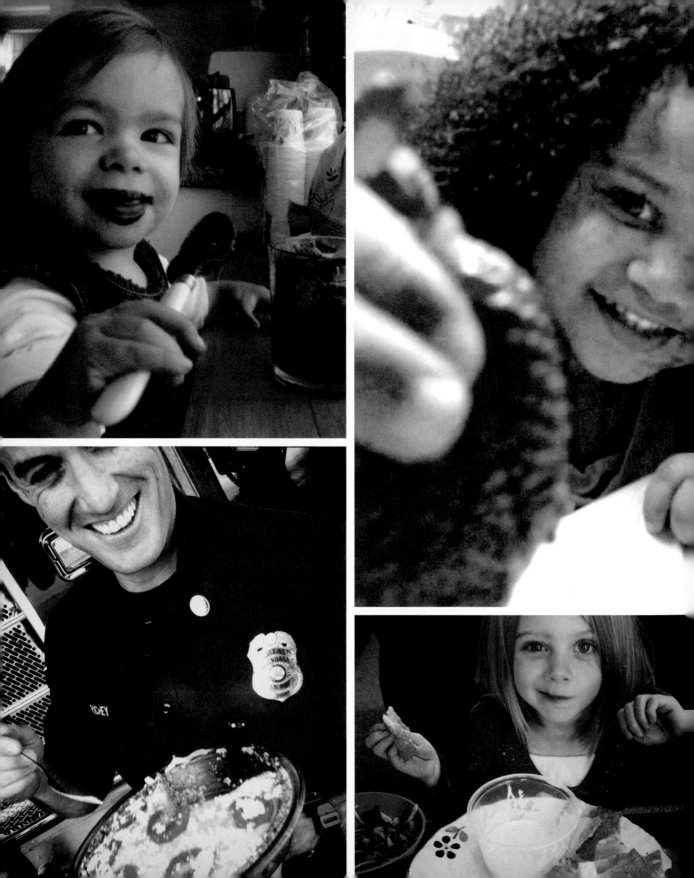

Contributors

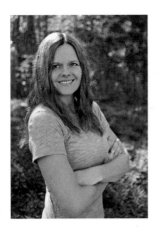

Thank you, Karen Nickel, my friend and absolutely amazingly talented photographer/foodie. Karen lives outside of Atlanta with her honey guy, Shawn, and two boys, Ocean and North. I came to feed the Nickel family when Karen found her own health concerns challenging and wanted to revamp her diet. We ate, we laughed, we mountain climbed (literally to my discomfort) and we took a lot of amazing photos. Karen has embraced a whole new way of life in the kitchen by starting her own website dedicated to raw newbies everywhere, RawNewbie.com.

Eli Dagostino, let no one be fooled by your young years. To be photographed by you felt special, intimate, funny, and a privilege. You truly caught my flavor. Thank you for my lifestyle photos. Here is to many more Happy Shakes together!

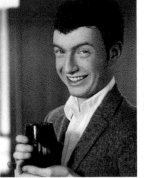

Photograph by Eli Dagostino

Acknowledgments

. . . THE MOST IMPORTANT!

Thank you, families, all my amazing families, each and every one of you for giving me the thousands on top of thousands of hours of education, from how to work my computer to my much developed mad skills in the kitchen. You have helped build in me so much confidence. I'm an expert all because of YOU! This book is dedicated to you and all my families I've yet to meet. Thank you!!!!!

Thank you, spinach, romaine, and broccoli. You have brought so much inspiration and delight to me and my families. Who knew you were so wonderful?!!

I must give a special thank you to CHOCOLATE. For so many years I thought you were bad news for me . . . a guilty pleasure. You are the closest thing to love in a food substance I have ever met. You got me through those early days stepping into raw food. You gave me hope. I love spreading your love. Thank you xoxo.

Thank you, Elizabeth Champion and Becky LeBlanc. From the West Coast to the East Coast, you both have kept me organized and sane. Thank you for heading up the test kitchens, and testing every single recipe until I got it all just right!

Thank you, Rebecca Avellino, for hair and makeup. You have taught me well and continue to keep me beautified. You are every little girl's dream!

Thank you, Chief Shivers and the Forsyth County Fire Department, for letting me feed you all and for taking the perfect picture of the Firehouse Tostadas! Thank you, Ken Iscol, Jill Iscol, Skip Bettencourt, and Nancy Hugger for your spectacular properties on Martha's Vineyard. The days with you made for the best photo ops and a lot of Happy Shake fun! Thank you to my models, Grace Segars, North Nickel, and Trevor White. Your warm smiles made those chilly days fun! Thank you, Liquiteria, my favorite Manhattan juice bar, for keeping us always juiced up!!!

To Louise Burke and all of my friends at Simon & Schuster, I feel so fortunate to have the finest, most skilled book people available to me. Thank you for all your hard work, expertise, and for letting me feed you along the way.

Thank you Trish for your sharp-eyed editing. You really know how to make a spell-check girl look good! Thank you for spending time with me, letting me feed you, and you feeding me your supportive excitement and energy. It truly was serendipity that we were brought together.

Jen Bergstrom, you are talented, tough, supportive, and enthusiastic . . . everything I would hope for in a publisher! But most important, thank you for being my friend. I love you.

Thank you, my dear husband, for your continued love and support. Thank you for getting my passion and love for families everywhere. Thank you for sitting me down to type my first words. Thank you for that safe quiet place you provide. I love you. I love you. I love you.

Index

Index

Index